Osteoporosis

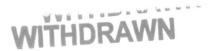

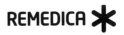
REMEDICA ✳

Published by Remedica
Commonwealth House, 1 New Oxford Street, London, WC1A 1NU, UK
Civic Opera Building, 20 North Wacker Drive, Suite 1642, Chicago, IL 60606, USA

info@remedicabooks.com
www.remedicabooks.com
Tel: +44 20 7759 2900
Fax: +44 20 7759 2951

Publisher: Andrew Ward
In-house editors: Carolyn Dunn, Cath Harris, Lyndsey Parker
Design and artwork: AS&K Skylight Creative Services

Previously published as 'Osteoporosis Illustrated'.

Remedica is a member of the AS&K Media Partnership.

ISBN-13: 978 1 850092 05 2
ISBN-10: 1 850092 05 2

British Library Cataloguing-in-Publication Data
A catalogue record for this book is available from the British Library.

Printed in Malta.

Osteoporosis

Nigel Arden, Editor
Senior Lecturer in Rheumatology
Medical Research Council Environmental Epidemiology Unit
University of Southampton
Southampton General Hospital
Southampton
UK

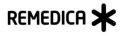

Contents

Contributors

Nigel Arden
Senior Lecturer in Rheumatology
Medical Research Council
Environmental Epidemiology Unit
University of Southampton
Southampton General Hospital
Southampton, UK

Ajay Bhatia
Specialist Registrar
Metabolic Bone Unit
The Royal National Orthopaedic Hospital
Stanmore, UK

Glen Blake
Senior Lecturer
Department of Nuclear Medicine
Guy's, King's and St Thomas' School of Medicine
London, UK

Pam Brown
General Practitioner
Swansea, UK

Judith Bubbear
Clinical Research Fellow
Metabolic Bone Unit
The Royal National Orthopaedic Hospital
Stanmore, UK

Jackie Clowes
ARC Clinical Scientist
Mayo Clinic and Foundation
Endocrine Research Unit
St Mary's Hospital
Rochester, MN, USA

Juliet Compston
Reader and Honorary Consultant Physician
Department of Medicine
Addenbrooke's Hospital
Cambridge, UK

Cyrus Cooper
Professor of Rheumatology
Medical Research Council
Environmental Epidemiology Unit
University of Southampton
Southampton General Hospital
Southampton, UK

Richard Eastell
Research Dean
Division of Clinical Sciences (North)
University of Sheffield
Northern General Hospital
Sheffield, UK

Ignac Fogelman
Professor of Nuclear Medicine
Department of Nuclear Medicine
Guy's, King's and St Thomas' School of Medicine
London, UK

Roger Francis
Reader in Medicine (Geriatrics)
Musculoskeletal Unit
Freeman Hospital
Newcastle upon Tyne, UK

Nicholas Harvey
Specialist Registrar
Medical Research Council
Environmental Epidemiology Unit
University of Southampton
Southampton General Hospital
Southampton, UK

Richard Keen
Consultant Rheumatologist
University College London
Centre for Rheumatology
London, UK

Ramasamyiyer Swaminathan
Professor of Clinical Chemistry
Department of Clinical Chemistry
Guy's, King's and St Thomas' School of Medicine
London, UK

Steve Tuck
Consultant Rheumatologist
James Cook University Hospital
Middlesbrough, UK

Introduction

Since the first edition of *Osteoporosis Illustrated* was published in 1997, knowledge about the causes and treatment of osteoporosis has continued to expand at a dramatic rate. There have been major advances in cellular biology, which have allowed further insights to be obtained into the pathogenesis of osteoporosis, and potentially two new therapeutic agents. There is now an ever-increasing array of techniques to measure bone density and size, which have helped to provide a greater understanding of the forces which affect bone fragility, including bone architecture and micro-architecture, as well as bone mineral density. Finally, there have been a number of new therapeutic agents on the market since the first edition, which have allowed more effective management of patients at high risk for osteoporotic fractures. This explosion of research has exponentially increased the amount of information available to clinicians via increasing numbers of dedicated osteoporosis journals and conferences in every country.

Most large text books are rapidly out of date in this fast moving field, and it is now difficult for even the most dedicated specialist to remain abreast of scientific and therapeutic advances. In this book, experts in their field have each provided a current 'state of the art' overview of the important areas in osteoporosis today. The style of the chapters, with figures and illustrations, is designed to facilitate understanding of the concepts and processes involved, in addition to providing an enjoyable read. Osteoporosis is now a treatable disease, let us hope we can all keep up with the advances going forward.

Nigel Arden
Editor

1

The Epidemiology of Osteoporotic Fractures

Nicholas Harvey and Cyrus Cooper

Definition of osteoporosis

Osteoporosis is a skeletal disease characterized by low bone mass and microarchitectural deterioration of bone tissue, with a consequent increase in bone fragility and susceptibility to fracture [1]. It is a major public health issue, affecting a large proportion of the population >50 years of age. It leads to a huge burden through the increased morbidity and mortality associated with fragility fractures.

The term 'osteoporosis' was first introduced in France and Germany in the 19th century. It means 'porous bone' and initially implied a histologic diagnosis, but was later refined to mean bone that was normally mineralized, but reduced in quantity (**Figure 1.1**).

The definition of osteoporosis has, historically, been difficult. A definition based on bone mineral density (BMD) might not encompass all of the risk factors for fracture, whereas a fracture-based definition will not enable the identification of

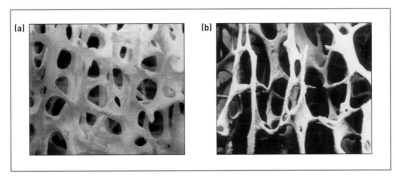

Figure 1.1 (a) Normal and **(b)** osteoporotic bone.

1

Definition	Criteria
Normal	BMC or BMD value <1.0 SD below the young normal mean
Low bone mass (osteopenia)	BMC or BMD value 1–2.5 SD below the young normal mean
Osteoporosis	BMC or BMD value >2.5 SD below the young normal mean
Established osteoporosis	Osteoporosis (see above) with one or more fragility fractures

Table 1.1 World Health Organization (WHO) classification of osteoporosis. Adapted from the WHO Study Group [2]. BMC: bone mineral content; BMD: bone mineral density; SD: standard deviation.

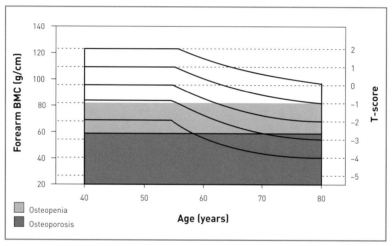

Figure 1.2 World Health Organization (WHO) definition of osteoporosis. BMC: bone mineral content.

at-risk populations. The World Health Organization has resolved this issue by defining osteoporosis in terms of BMD and previous fracture, as shown in **Table 1.1** and **Figure 1.2** [2].

If this definition is applied to a female population sample in the UK, the prevalence of osteoporosis at the femoral neck rises from 5.1% at age 50–54 years to >60% at age ≥85 years. The corresponding estimates for men are 0.4% and 29.1%, respectively.

All fractures

Data from the UK suggest that there is an overall fracture incidence of 21.1/1,000 per year (23.5/1,000 men and 18.8/1,000 women) [3] and that there

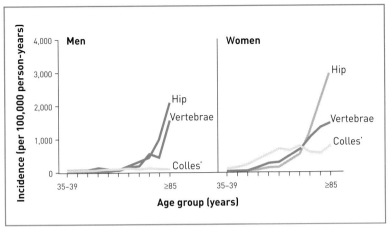

Figure 1.3 Age-specific incidence rates for hip, vertebral, and Colles' fractures. Reproduced with permission from Elsevier [5].

is a bimodal distribution, with peaks in youth and in the very elderly [4]. Fractures of long bones predominate in young people, usually as a result of substantial trauma, and males are more frequently involved than females. Thus, it is the magnitude of the trauma, rather than deficient bone strength, that leads to the fracture in this group. In the elderly, low bone mass is the critical factor, with most fractures occurring as a result of minimal force. The rate of fracture in women increases steeply after the age of 35 years, and becomes twice that in men **(Figure 1.3)** [5].

Hip and distal forearm fractures are the main contributors to this peak, which also includes proximal humeral, pelvic, and proximal tibial fractures. A study from Denmark showed that 60-year-old women, expected to live until the age of 81 years, had an estimated residual lifetime risk of radial, humeral, or hip fracture of 17%, 8%, and 14%, respectively. The lifetime risk to women surviving to the age of 88 years was increased to 32% [6]. There are site-specific differences in fracture risk related to age and sex; these will be detailed in the following sections.

Hip fracture

Hip fracture is the most devastating consequence of osteoporosis, invariably requiring hospitalization. Typically, hip fractures result from a fall from standing height or less, but may occur spontaneously [7]. The diagnosis is usually suggested by characteristic clinical features, and confirmed by a plain radiograph. Fractures are classified as intracapsular (through the femoral neck) or extracapsular **(Figure 1.4)**.

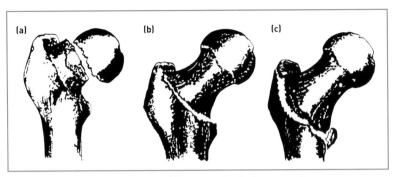

Figure 1.4 Classification of hip fractures. (a) intracapsular, (b,c) extracapsular.

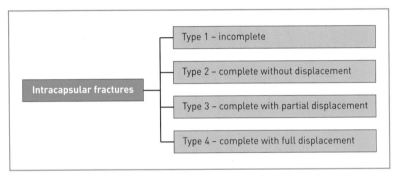

Figure 1.5 Classification of intracapsular fractures according to the Garden scale.

Intracapsular fractures are usually classified according to the Garden scale (**Figure 1.5**). Extracapsular fractures are intertrochanteric or subtrochanteric, and are classified as stable or unstable, and according to displacement (**Figure 1.6**).

The classification of a fracture has important implications for its orthopedic management, as the blood supply to the femoral head is precarious and liable to compromise with certain patterns of fracture. There were an estimated 1.66 million hip fractures worldwide in 1990: 1,197,000 in women and 463,000 in men [8].

Impact
Hip fracture is the most devastating manifestation of osteoporosis: 5–20% of people will die within 1 year of a hip fracture, and >50% of survivors will be incapacitated, many needing nursing-home care (**Table 1.2**).

Mortality
The majority of excess deaths occur within 6 months of the fracture and diminish with time so that, after 2 years, survival is comparable with that of similarly

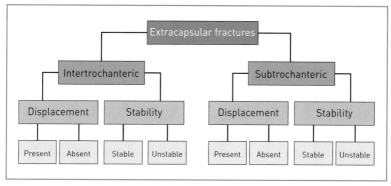

Figure 1.6 Classification of extracapsular fractures.

Time from diagnosis (years)	Vertebral	Hip	Forearm
1	0.88 (0.85–0.91)	0.96 (0.92–0.99)	1.00 (0.98–1.02)
2	0.87 (0.83–0.90)	0.93 (0.87–0.99)	1.00 (0.97–1.03)
3	0.86 (0.82–0.90)	0.92 (0.86–0.98)	1.01 (0.98–1.04)
4	0.83 (0.78–0.88)	0.84 (0.75–0.92)	0.99 (0.95–1.04)
5	0.83 (0.77–0.89)	0.82 (0.71–0.93)	1.00 (0.95–1.05)

Table 1.2 Relative survival (95% confidence interval) following vertebral, hip, and distal forearm fractures among residents of Rochester, MN, USA, according to duration of follow-up from diagnosis. Data from Cooper and Melton [5].

aged men and women in the general population. Mortality differs, however, according to the age and gender of the person experiencing the hip fracture. In a population-based study, a relative survival rate of 92% was found for white hip-fracture victims <75 years of age, compared with 83% in those aged ≥75 years at the time of the fracture [9]. Despite their greater age at the time of fracture, survival was better among women.

This gender difference has been confirmed in other hospital-based studies and appears to be due to the greater frequency of other chronic diseases in men who sustain hip fractures. The majority of deaths after hip fracture are due to pre-existing co-morbidity, such as ischemic heart disease, with the minority being a direct result of complications or management of the fracture itself.

Morbidity
In the USA, 7% of survivors of all types of fracture have some degree of permanent disability, and 8% require long-term nursing-home care. Overall, a 50-year-old white American woman has a 13% chance of experiencing

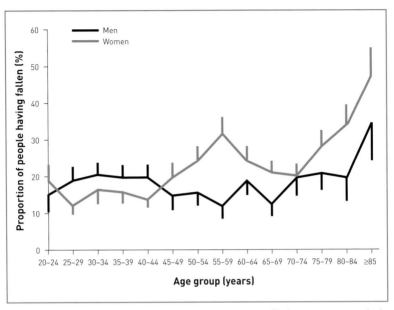

Figure 1.7 Proportion of people reporting a fall in the previous year. The bars represent standard errors. Data from Winner et al [12].

functional decline after any fracture [10]. As with mortality, hip fractures contribute most to osteoporosis-associated disability. Patients are prone to developing acute complications such as pressure sores, bronchopneumonia, and urinary tract infections. Perhaps the most important long-term outcome is impairment of the ability to walk. Fifty per cent of those ambulatory before the fracture are unable to walk independently afterwards. Age is an important determinant of outcome, with 14% of 50- to 55-year-old hip-fracture victims being discharged to nursing homes, versus 55% of those >90 years old [10].

Determinants

Age
There is an exponential increase in hip fracture with aging (see **Figure 1.3**). This is due to an age-related increase in the risk of falling, and an age-related reduction in bone strength. The majority occur after a fall from standing height or less: 90% occur in people >50 years of age and 80% are in women [11]. Among postmenopausal women in the USA, the likelihood of experiencing at least one fall annually rises from about one in five women aged 60–64 years of age to one in three women aged 80–84 years [7]. Comparable data were found in the UK (**Figure 1.7**), with one in three women aged 80–84 years having fallen in the previous year; this rose to nearly 50% in women aged ≥85 years [12].

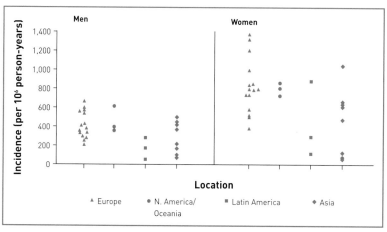

Figure 1.8 Hip-fracture incidence around the world. Data from Kanis et al [17].

One-third of men in the oldest age group experienced a fall in the preceding year. However, only about 1% of all falls lead to a hip fracture. This is because the amount of trauma delivered to the proximal femur depends upon various protective responses and the orientation of the fall – falling sideways onto the hip is more likely to result in fracture than falling forwards [13].

Femoral neck strength is weaker in women than in men and declines with age in both sexes. Many factors contribute to bone strength (eg, BMD and microarchitecture), but all are closely correlated with absolute bone mass. Over a lifetime, the BMD of the femoral neck declines an estimated 58% in women and 39% in men, while bone density of the intertrochanteric region of the proximal femur falls by about 53% and 35%, respectively. Each one standard deviation decline in BMD is associated with a 1.8- to 2.6-fold increase in the age-adjusted risk of hip fracture, depending on the exact site that is measured [14].

Gender

The incidence of osteoporotic hip fractures is lower in men than in women. To illustrate, in 1990 only about 30% of 1.66 million hip fractures worldwide occurred in men [15]. Men are relatively protected for several reasons: they have a higher peak density, they lose less bone during aging, they do not become hypogonadal, they sustain fewer falls, and they have a shorter lifespan. However, this relationship is not true for all populations – in black and Asian groups, the incidence of hip fractures is slightly higher in men [16].

Ethnicity

Hip fractures are much more frequent among whites than among non-whites. This has been explained by the higher bone mass observed in blacks compared with whites **(Figure 1.8)** [17].

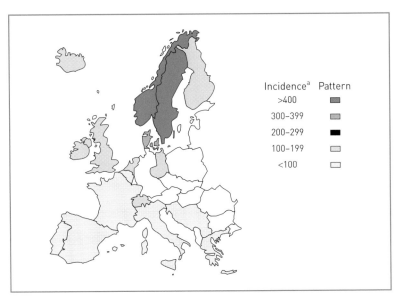

Figure 1.9 European incidence of hip fracture in females. Data from Elffors et al, Johnell et al, and Nagant de Deuxchaisnes and Devogelaer [22–24]. [a]Crude rate/10,000 of the population ≥50 years.

There is also some evidence that the rate of bone loss is lower in blacks. However, the Bantu people of South Africa have lower fracture rates than whites and a lower bone mass [18]. Likewise, the incidence of hip fractures among women of Japanese ancestry is about half that of their white counterparts, even though their bone mass is somewhat lower [19]. These discrepancies may be related to a lower frequency of falls, as a lower risk of falling has been reported among black women compared with white women [20]. Asian women have shorter femoral necks than white women, and this shape seems inherently less likely to fracture, despite a lower BMD [21].

Geography

There is variation in the incidence of hip fracture within populations of a given race and gender **(Figure 1.9)** [22–24]. Thus, age-adjusted hip-fracture incidence rates are higher among white residents of Scandinavia than comparable subjects in the USA or Oceania. In 1986, the Mediterranean Osteoporosis Study (MEDOS) was set up to investigate the incidence of hip fracture in the Mediterranean region. It was discovered that the incidence of hip fracture varied markedly from country to country, and even within countries. Within Europe, the range of variation was approximately 11-fold [22]. These differences were not explained by variation in activity levels, smoking, obesity, alcohol consumption, or migration status [23]. The geographic differences in the UK were not associated with differences in water fluoridation or with dietary calcium intake, as assessed by a national food survey [25].

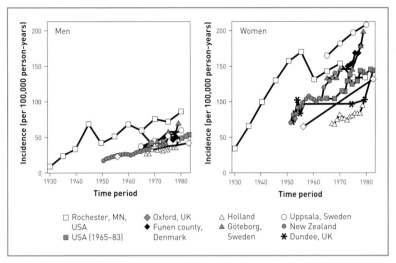

Figure 1.10 Incidence of hip fractures over time as reported in various studies.
Adapted from Melton et al [29].

Studies in the USA confirm this complex pattern. In over 2,000 counties nationwide, the age-adjusted incidence of hip fracture in white women aged >65 years of age was negatively associated with latitude (higher in the south), water hardness, and hours of January sunlight, and positively associated with poverty levels, proportion of the land in farms, and proportion of the population with fluoridated water [26].

Season
Hip fractures are seasonal, occurring more frequently during the winter in temperate countries in both men and women. However, the majority of hip fractures follow falls indoors and are not related to slipping on icy surfaces. Explanations for this include abnormal neuromuscular function at lower temperatures and a winter reduction in sunlight exposure, with consequent vitamin D deficiency.

Time trends
Life expectancy is increasing around the globe and the number of elderly individuals is rising in every geographic region. There are currently 323 million individuals aged ≥65 years, and this number is expected to reach 1,555 million by the year 2050. These demographic changes alone can be expected to increase the number of hip fractures occurring among people aged ≥35 years throughout the world; the incidence is estimated to rise from 1.66 million in 1990 to 6.26 million in 2050. Assuming a constant age-specific rate of fracture, as the number of people aged >65 years increases from 32 million in 1990 to 69 million in 2050, the number of hip fractures in the USA will increase 3-fold [27]. In the UK,

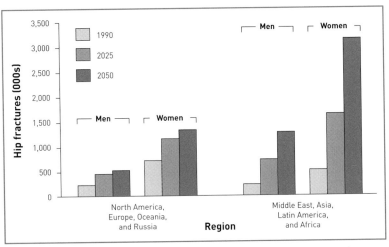

Figure 1.11 Estimated numbers of hip fractures among men and women in different regions of the world in 1990 and 2050. Data from Cooper et al [27].

the number of hip fractures is projected to increase from 46,000 in 1985 to 117,000 in 2016 [28]. **Figure 1.10** summarizes the results from several studies [29].

An increasingly elderly population in Latin America and Asia could lead to a shift in the geographic distribution of hip fractures, with only a quarter occurring in Europe and North America (**Figure 1.11**) [27].

Such projections may be deemed optimistic considering that increases in the incidence of hip fractures have been observed, even after adjusting for the growth in the elderly population. Although the age-adjusted rate of hip fracture appears to have leveled off in the northern regions of the USA, parts of Sweden, and the UK, the rates in Hong Kong rose substantially between 1966 and 1985. Thus, the above figures potentially represent a significant underestimate of the number of hip fractures in the next half-century.

There are three broad explanations for these trends:

- Firstly, they might represent some increasingly prevalent current risk factor for osteoporosis or falling; physical activity is the most likely candidate. There is ample evidence linking inactivity to the risk of hip fracture, whether this effect is mediated through bone density, the risk of falls, or both. Furthermore, some of the steepest secular trends have been observed in Asian countries, such as Hong Kong, which have witnessed dramatic reductions in the customary activity levels of their populations in recent decades.
- The second explanation is that the elderly population is becoming increasingly frail. As many of the disorders leading to frailty are independently associated

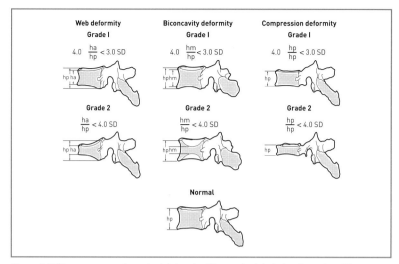

Figure 1.12 Measurements of vertebral deformity. SD: standard deviation. Reproduced from *J Bone Miner Res* 1991;6:207–15 with permission of the American Society for Bone and Mineral Research [31].

with osteoporosis and the risk of falling, this tendency might have contributed to the secular increases in western nations during earlier decades of this century.

- Finally, the trends could arise from a cohort phenomenon – some adverse influence on bone mass or the risk of falling that acted at an earlier time and is now manifesting as a rising incidence of fractures in successive generations of the elderly.

Vertebral fracture

Definition

Vertebral fractures have been synonymous with the diagnosis of osteoporosis since its earliest description as a metabolic bone disorder [30]. However, knowledge of its epidemiology remains scant because there is no universally accepted definition of a vertebral fracture from thoracolumbar radiographs, and because a substantial proportion of vertebral deformities are asymptomatic.

The difficulty in deciding whether a vertebral body is deformed results from the variation in the shape of vertebrae, both within the spine and between individuals. Early epidemiologic studies of vertebral fractures used subjective radiologic assessments of wedge, crush, and biconcave deformities, but these were poorly reproducible. These methods gave way to morphometric measurements of vertebral height, with fractures defined according to fixed cut-off values (**Figure 1.12**).

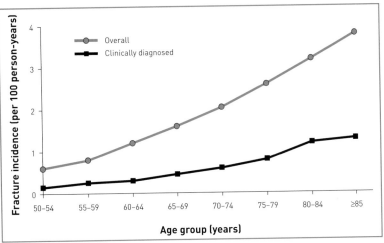

Figure 1.13 The incidence of vertebral deformities in a population sample of women from the USA. Data from Cooper et al [8].

However, each vertebral body in the spinal column has unique dimensions, and analyses have focused on determining the distribution of vertebral dimensions at each spinal level and calculating cut-off values from these [31,32]. The most widely adopted thresholds for defining and grading deformities are:

- Moderate (grade 1) fractures which are deformities that fall between three and four standard deviations from the mean value specific to each vertebra.
- Severe (grade 2) fractures which are those that fall four standard deviations or more from this mean.

When morphometric studies are performed without reference to clinical presentation, the abnormalities found are usually referred to as deformities rather than fractures. Three broad categories of vertebral fracture have been described:

- compression (crush) fractures, where there is loss of both anterior and posterior vertebral height
- wedge (partial) fractures, where anterior height tends to be lost
- biconcave (balloon) fractures, where loss of central bony tissue leads to concavity of both vertebral end plates

Incidence and prevalence

Incidence

The application of recently developed morphometric techniques to various population samples in the USA has permitted the estimation of the incidence of new vertebral fractures in the general population (**Figure 1.13**).

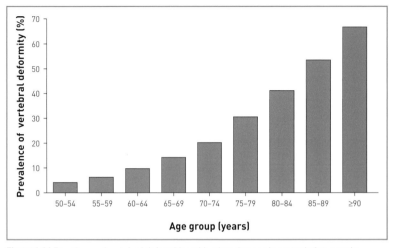

Figure 1.14 Prevalence of vertebral deformities with advancing age in a population sample of women from Rochester, MN, USA. Data from Melton et al [35].

Using the data shown, the age-adjusted incidence among white US women aged ≥50 years was found to be 18 per 1,000 person-years [33]. This is more than twice the corresponding incidence of hip fracture (6.2 per 1,000 person-years). It is important to note the disparity between the incidence of vertebral fractures identified on radiographs and those reported clinically. In Rochester, MN, USA, the incidence of clinically diagnosed vertebral deformities was 30% of that expected from a study using radiographic diagnosis. This implies that two thirds of vertebral fractures do not come to medical attention [8]. A similar study using the General Practice Research Database (GPRD), which covers 6% of the UK population, suggested that the figure may be nearer to 90% [34].

Prevalence
The prevalence of vertebral deformity was investigated in an age-stratified random sample of the population of Rochester. The prevalence was estimated at 25.3 per 100 Rochester women aged ≥50 years (95% confidence interval 22.3–28.2) **(Figure 1.14)** [35].

Data from a large European study (EVOS [European Vertebral Osteoporosis Study]) suggested less variation in the prevalence of vertebral fracture across European countries than is apparent for hip fracture [36].

Impact
Vertebral fractures cause significant pain, deformity, and long-term disability. Data from the Study of Osteoporotic Fractures, a US population-based study of 9,606 women aged ≥65 years, showed that women who had grade 2 deformities were 2.6 times more likely to suffer disability and 1.9 times more likely to report

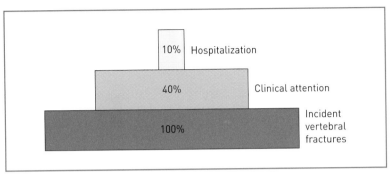

Figure 1.15 Overall outcome of vertebral fractures. Data from Cooper et al [8].

moderate or severe back pain than those with no deformity [37]. Women with grade 1 deformities did not have significantly elevated risks of these clinical sequelae. Cross-sectional data from out-patients also support this notion, with severe vertebral deformity being much more closely associated with adverse outcomes than moderate deformity [38]. **Figure 1.15** shows the overall outcome of vertebral fractures.

Mortality
Examination of the survival of patients following a clinically diagnosed vertebral fracture rather surprisingly reveals a similar excess mortality at 5 years to that found with hip fractures **(Figure 1.16)**. This excess is observed in patients with vertebral fractures caused by moderate or minimal trauma, but not in those whose fractures follow severe trauma.

The impairment of survival following vertebral fracture also markedly worsens as time from diagnosis of the fracture increases. This is in contrast to the pattern of survival for hip fractures. Furthermore, there does not appear to be any particular cause of death that explains this finding. This accords with the observations of US and Swedish studies that low bone density *per se* is associated with premature death [39,40]. These data suggest that the association might be due to a number of factors, such as smoking, alcohol consumption, and immobility; these predispose independently to both bone loss and death.

Morbidity
The health impact of vertebral fractures has proved to be considerably difficult to quantify. As stated earlier, only a minority of vertebral deformities come to the attention of clinicians. Nonetheless, vertebral fractures in patients aged ≥45 years account for 52,000 hospital admissions in the USA and 2,188 in England and Wales each year. The major clinical consequences of vertebral fractures are back pain, kyphosis, and height loss. New compression fractures may give rise to severe back pain, which typically decreases in severity over several weeks or months. This pain is associated with exquisite localized

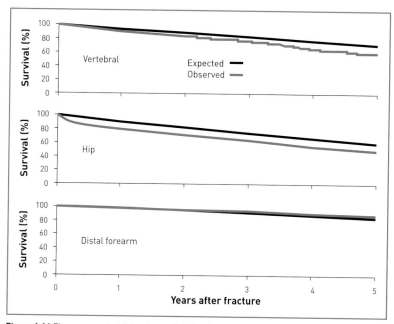

Figure 1.16 Five-year survival following a clinically diagnosed hip, vertebral, or distal forearm fracture in Rochester, MN, USA, 1985–1989. Reproduced with permission from Oxford University Press [33].

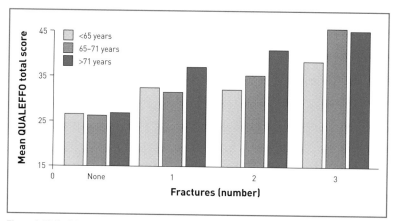

Figure 1.17 Health-related quality of life related to age and number of vertebral deformities. QUALEFFO: Quality of Life Questionaire of the European Foundation for Osteoporosis. Reproduced from *J Bone Miner Res* 2000;15:1384–92 with permission of the American Society for Bone and Mineral Research [41].

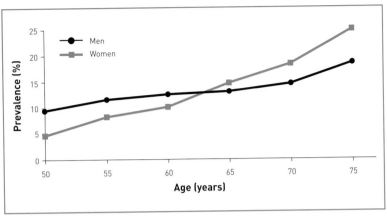

Figure 1.18 Prevalence of vertebral deformity. Data from O'Neill et al [36].

tenderness and paravertebral muscle spasm, which markedly limits spinal movements. **Figure 1.17** shows QUALEFFO (Quality of Life Questionnaire of the European Foundation for Osteoporosis) score against age and number of vertebral fractures [41]. This clearly shows the impact of age and number of fractures, with higher QUALEFFO scores indicating lower health-related quality of life.

A more protracted clinical course affects a proportion of patients with a history of chronic pain experienced while standing and during physical stress, particularly bending. For example, in the control group of one treatment study, patients were noted to have persistent pain for 6 months following fracture [42]. This chronic pain is thought to arise from spinal extensor muscle weakness, as well as the altered spinal biomechanics, which result from vertebral deformation. A number of indices of physical function, self-esteem, body image, and mood also appear to be adversely affected in patients with vertebral fractures. Whenever self-report scales of functional status or quality of life have been applied to patients with vertebral fractures, scores are found to be worse for those with more severe or multiple deformities [43].

Determinants

Age
Most studies concur that the prevalence of vertebral fractures rises with age among women. **Figure 1.14** shows that, in an age-stratified random sample of 762 Rochester women who underwent thoracolumbar radiography, the prevalence of one or more deformities increased from 7.6% at age 50–54 years to 64.3% in those aged ≥90 years.

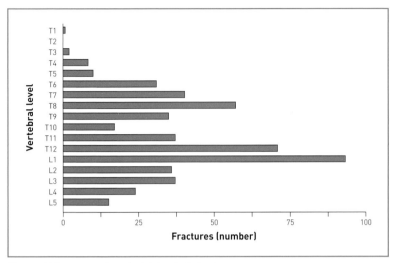

Figure 1.19 Prevalence of vertebral deformity by level.

Figure 1.3 shows the incidence rates of clinically diagnosed vertebral fractures in men and women. In men, incidence climbs exponentially with age, adopting a pattern similar to that observed for hip fractures in the same population. In women, there is a more linear increase in incidence with age, such that vertebral fracture rates are higher than those for hip fractures before the age of 70 years, but not thereafter.

Gender

Although it is generally believed that vertebral fracture is much more common in women than in men, there is little epidemiologic evidence to support this notion. The incidence of vertebral fractures in men appears to be low at around 1–2 per 1,000 per year. However, examination of limited regions of the spine, variable definitions of what constitutes a fracture, and incomplete case ascertainment have made it difficult to provide a stable and reliable assessment of vertebral fracture incidence and prevalence in men. Most of the prevalence studies conducted have been confined to women, and the few to include men have produced inconsistent results [44,45].

Figure 1.3 illustrates that male vertebral fractures are a greater problem than has previously been recognized, with an overall age-adjusted incidence in women only 1.9 times greater than in men [8]. Most recently, the results of EVOS have shown that, overall, men aged 50–64 years have a higher prevalence of deformity compared with similarly aged women, with the reverse being the case for those aged ≥65 years **(Figure 1.18)** [36]. Whereas 90% of vertebral fractures in women occurred as a result of moderate or minimal trauma in this study, an appreciable

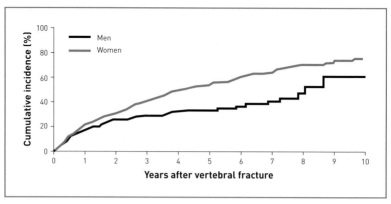

Figure 1.20 Risk of subsequent fracture after initial vertebral fracture. Data from Melton et al [48].

proportion of those in men (37%) occurred as a result of severe trauma, eg, road traffic accidents.

The most frequent vertebral levels involved are Ll, T8, and T12 **(Figure 1.19)**. These correspond with the most biomechanically compromised regions of the thoracolumbar spine: the mid-thoracic region, where dorsal kyphosis is most pronounced, and the thoracolumbar junction, where the relatively rigid thoracic spine meets the freely moving lumbar segment.

Ethnicity
There are few studies assessing the influence of ethnicity on vertebral fracture prevalence, although one found vertebral deformities in around 5% of selected white women aged ≥45 years, but in none of 137 black women studied [46]. This finding is in accord with the often-replicated observation that hip-fracture incidence rates are markedly higher among whites. However, data from Japan suggest that prevalence rates for vertebral deformity in Oriental women may be similar to those observed in white populations [47].

Previous fracture
A prevalent vertebral deformity increases the risk of subsequent fractures significantly. This is explored further in **Chapter 3**, but **Figure 1.20** summarizes the cumulative incidence of a subsequent vertebral fracture over time after a baseline event [48].

Time trends
The impact of osteoporotic fractures is set to rise in the future, commensurate with the increasing number of elderly people in the population. Little is known about secular increases in the age-adjusted incidence of vertebral fractures. In Rochester, there was no significant increase in the incidence of clinically diagnosed vertebral fractures between 1950 and 1989 [49]. However, when

categorized into subgroups, a significant increase in the incidence of fractures following moderate or minimal trauma in postmenopausal women is revealed. This increase occurred between 1950 and 1964, with a plateau in age-adjusted incidence thereafter. Rates for severe trauma fractures, and for vertebral fractures from any cause among younger men and women, remained stable. This rise in moderate trauma fractures in women paralleled that for hip fractures in Rochester. An increase in the prevalence of osteoporosis over this period is compatible with these trends.

Two European studies have also investigated secular trends in the incidence of vertebral fractures. Men and women, aged ≥60 years, presenting with thoracic and lumbar vertebral fractures between 1950 and 1952, and 1982 and 1983, in Malmo, Sweden, were studied [50]. Among women, incidence rates during 1982–83 were higher than those during 1950–52 at all ages >60 years. Among men, the increase was only apparent at >80 years. The prevalence of radiographic vertebral deformities in two samples of 70-year-old Danish women studied in 1979 and 1989 were found to be virtually identical [51]. The secular tendency reported from Rochester, with a rise in incidence between 1950 and 1964, followed by a plateau, is consistent with both of these reports.

Geography
The EVOS study found a 3-fold difference in the prevalence of vertebral deformities between countries, with the highest rates in Scandinavia. The prevalence range between centers was 7.5–19.8% for men and 6.2–20.7% for women. The differences were not as great as those seen for hip fracture in Europe, and some of the differences could be explained by levels of physical activity and body mass index.

Distal forearm fracture

Definition
Distal forearm fractures nearly always follow a fall on an outstretched arm. The most common distal forearm fracture is Colles' fracture. This fracture lies within 2.5 cm of the wrist joint margin. It is associated with dorsal angulation and displacement of the distal fragment of the radius, and with fracture of the ulnar styloid **(Figure 1.21)** [52].

Impact
Despite the fact that only around one-fifth of all patients with distal forearm fractures are hospitalized, they account for some 50,000 hospital admissions and over 400,000 physician visits in the USA each year, and 10,000 hospital admissions in the UK. Admission rates appear to vary markedly with age, such that only 16% of those occurring in women aged 45–54 years of age require in-patient care, compared with 76% of those occurring in women aged ≥85 years. There is a 30% increase of algodystrophy after these fractures, as well as a risk of neuropathies and posttraumatic arthritis. Wrist fractures do not

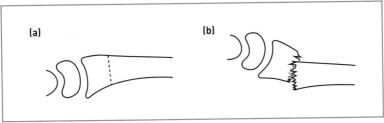

Figure 1.21 Fracture of the distal radius. **(a)** A normal wrist (lateral view). **(b)** Colles' fracture, with the characteristic dorsal angulation of the distal radius. Reproduced with permission from Elsevier [52].

appear to increase mortality. Although wrist fractures have an impact on some activities such as writing or meal preparation, overall, few patients are completely disabled, despite over half reporting only fair to poor function at 6 months [10,53,54].

Determinants

Age
Distal forearm fractures display a different pattern of incidence to that of the other osteoporotic fractures (see **Figure 1.3**). In white women, incidence rates increase linearly between 40 and 65 years of age, and then stabilize. In men, the incidence remains constant between 20 and 80 years. The reason for the plateau in female incidence remains obscure, but could relate to a change in the pattern of falling with advancing age. The slower gait and impaired neuromuscular coordination of elderly women makes them more likely to fall on their hip rather than on their wrist. However, more recent studies have shown a gentle progressive increase in incidence after the menopause [55], suggesting that there has been a change in the pattern of incidence with age, the explanation for which is not clear.

Gender
The age-adjusted female to male ratio of 4:1 for distal forearm fractures is more marked than either hip or vertebral fractures. Fifty per cent occur in women >65 years of age. After the age of 35 years, the age-adjusted incidence of wrist fracture is 36.8 per 10,000 person-years in women and 9.0 per 10,000 person-years in men. The incidence in men is low and does not markedly rise with aging [56].

Season
There is a winter peak in the incidence of Colles' fracture. This peak is more pronounced than that observed in hip fracture, and is also more closely related to falls outdoors during episodes of icy weather. This seasonal variation has been found in northern Europe, but is not apparent in southern Europe.

	Hip	Spine	Wrist
Lifetime risk (%)			
Women	14	11	13
Men	3	2	2
Cases/year	400,000	270,000	330,000
Hospitalization (%)	100	2–10	25
Relative survival	0.83	0.82	1.00
Costs: All sites combined ~ €17 billion			

Table 1.3 Impact of osteoporosis-related fractures in Europe. From Cooper [59].

Cost of osteoporotic fractures

The total cost of osteoporosis is difficult to assess because it includes in-patient and out-patient medical care, loss of working days, chronic nursing-home costs, and medication. The direct costs of osteoporosis stem mainly from the management of patients with hip fractures.

In the UK, hip-fracture patients occupy one-fifth of all orthopedic beds. In 1994, the direct cost in England and Wales was £750 million [57], and a more recent estimate puts the figure at £942 million [58]. In France, an estimated 56,000 hip fractures annually cost about €0.5 billion. The cost of fractures in the USA may be as much as $20 billion per year, with hip fractures accounting for over one-third of the total. **Table 1.3** summarizes the impact of osteoporotic fractures in Europe in the 1990s, reaching a total cost of around €17 billion [59]. **Table 1.4** illustrates that the greatest expense is incurred by the in-patient, out-patient, and nursing-home care of hip fractures [60].

Based on the outcome probabilities shown in **Table 1.5**, it can be estimated that 10% of women who sustain a hip fracture become functionally dependent in the activities of daily living (taking pre-fracture functional status into account), and that 19% require long-term nursing-home care because of the fracture.

Nursing-home care is extremely expensive, accounting for over half of the total annual cost of hip fractures. At least 60,000 nursing-home admissions are attributed to hip fractures each year in the USA. As many as 8% of all nursing-home residents have had a hip fracture.

Type of cost	Cost ($m)
Direct costs	
Hospital in-patient services	3,077
Hospital out-patient services	778
Physician services	403
Other practitioner services	11
Drugs	5
Nursing-home care	1,565
Pre-payments and administration	339
Non-health sector goods and services	875
Indirect costs	
Morbidity	1,415
Mortality[a]	260
Total	8,728

Table 1.4 Estimated cost of hip fractures by type of cost, 1988. [a]Present value of lifetime earnings discounted at 4%. Data from Praemer et al [60].

Pre-fracture status	Independent	Dependent	Nursing-home
Independent	0.74	0.18	0.08
Dependent	–	0.50	0.50
Nursing-home	–	–	1.00

Table 1.5 Probability of post-hip fracture outcomes by pre-fracture functional status. Data from Chrischilles et al [10].

Fracture site	Steroid dose (mg)		
	<2.5	2.5–7.5	≥7.5
Nonvertebral	1.17 (1.10–1.25)	1.36 (1.28–1.43)	1.64 (1.54–1.76)
Hip	0.99 (0.82–1.20)	1.77 (1.55–2.02)	2.27 (1.94–2.66)
Radius/ulna	1.10 (0.96–1.25)	1.04 (0.93–1.17)	1.19 (1.02–1.39)
Vertebral	1.55 (1.20–2.01)	2.59 (2.16–3.10)	5.18 (4.25–6.31)

Table 1.6 Steroid dose and relative risk of fractures. Numbers in brackets give the 95% confidence interval. Reproduced from *J Bone Miner Res* 2000;15:993–1000 with permission of the American Society for Bone and Mineral Research [61].

Corticosteroid-induced osteoporosis

Osteoporosis can be primary, as in postmenopausal osteoporosis, or secondary to other factors, such as medication. Of all drugs, corticosteroids have some of the most adverse effects on bone health. Historically, it had been felt that there was a cut-off at around 7.5 mg prednisolone daily, below which fracture risk was not increased. However, work using the GPRD by van Staa et al has demonstrated unequivocally that there is no safe dose [61,62]. This is shown in **Table 1.6**. New guidelines on the prevention and treatment of corticosteroid-induced osteoporosis were published in 2002 [63].

Conclusion

Osteoporosis is a disease that has a huge effect on public health. The impact of osteoporotic fracture is massive, not just for individuals, but for health services, economies, and populations as a whole. Strategies to reduce the burden of this widespread disease are thus urgently needed.

References

1. Anon. Consensus development conference: diagnosis, prophylaxis and treatment of osteoporosis. *Am J Med* 1993;94:646–50.

2. Kanis JA. Assessment of fracture risk and its application to screening for postmenopausal osteoporosis: synopsis of a WHO report. WHO Study Group. *Osteoporos Int* 1994;4:368–81.

3. Johansen A, Evans RJ, Stone MD, et al. Fracture incidence in England and Wales: a study based on the population of Cardiff. *Injury* 1997;28:655–60.

4. Cooper C, O'Neill T, Silman A, on behalf of the European Vertebral Osteoporosis Study Group. The epidemiology of vertebral fractures. *Bone* 1993;14:S89–97.

5. Cooper C, Melton LJ III. Magnitude and impact of osteoporosis and fractures. In: Marcus R, Feldman O, Kelsey J, eds. *Osteoporosis*. San Diego: Academic Press Inc, 1996:419–34.

6. Lauritzen JB, Schwarz P, Lund B, et al. Changing incidence and residual lifetime risk of common osteoporosis-related fractures. *Osteoporos Int* 1993;3:127–32.

7. Nevitt MC, Cummings SR. Study of Osteoporotic Fractures Research Group. Type of fall and risk of hip and wrist fractures; the study of osteoporotic fractures. *J Am Geriatr Soc* 1993;41:1226–34.

8. Cooper C, Atkinson EJ, O'Fallon WM, et al. Incidence of clinically diagnosed vertebral fractures: a population-based study in Rochester, Minnesota, 1985–1989. *J Bone Miner Res* 1992;7:221–7.

9. Melton LJ III. Epidemiology of fractures. In: Riggs BL, Melton LJ III, eds. *Osteoporosis: Etiology, Diagnosis and Management*. New York: Raven Press, 1995:133–54.

10. Chrischilles EA, Butler CD, Davis CS, et al. A model of lifetime osteoporosis impact. *Arch Intern Med* 1991;151:2026–32.

11. Gallagher JC, Melton LJ III, Riggs BL, et al. Epidemiology of fractures of the proximal femur in Rochester, Minnesota. *Clin Orthop Rel Res* 1980;150:163–71.

12. Winner SJ, Morgan CA, Evans JG. Perimenopausal risk of falling and incidence of distal forearm fracture. *BMJ* 1989;298:1486–8.

13. Melton LJ III, Riggs BL. Risk factors for injury after a fall. *Clin Geriatr Med* 1985;1:525–39.

14. Marshall D, Johnell O, Wedel H. Meta-analysis of how well measures of bone mineral density predict occurrence of osteoporotic fractures. *BMJ* 1996;312:1254–9.

15. Anderson DC. Osteoporosis in men. *BMJ* 1992;305:489–90.

16. Garton MJ, Reid DM. Osteoporosis in the 1990s: investigation and management. *Hospital Update* 1993;6:363–7.

17. Kanis JA, Johnell O, De Laet C, et al. International variations in hip fracture probabilities: implications for risk assessment. *J Bone Miner Res* 2002;17:1237–44.

18. Solomon L. Bone density in aging Caucasian and African populations. *Lancet* 1979;2:1326–30.

19. Ross PD, Norimatsu H, Davis JW, et al. A comparison of hip fracture incidence among native Japanese, Japanese-Americans, and American Caucasians. *Am J Epidemiol* 1991;133:801–9.

20. Tinetti ME, Speechley M, Ginter SF. Risk factors for falls among elderly persons living in the community. *N Engl J Med* 1988;319:1701–7.

21. Cummings SR, Cauley JA, Palermo L, et al. Study of Osteoporotic Fractures Research Group. Racial differences in hip axis lengths might explain racial differences in rates of hip fracture. *Osteoporos Int* 1994;4:226–9.

22. Elffors I, Allander E, Kanis JA, et al. The variable incidence of hip fracture in southern Europe: the MEDOS study. *Osteoporos Int* 1994;4:253–63.

23. Johnell O, Gullberg B, Allander E, et al. The apparent incidence of hip fracture in Europe: a study of national register sources. *Osteoporos Int* 1992;2:298–302.

24. Nagant de Deuxchaisnes C, Devogelaer JP. Increase in the incidence of hip fracture and of the ratio of trochanteric to cervical hip fracture in Belgium. *Calcif Tissue Int* 1988;42:201–3.

25. Cooper C, Wickham C, Lacey RF, et al. Water fluoride concentration and fracture of the proximal femur. *J Epidemiol Community Health* 1990;44:17–19.

26. Jacobsen SJ, Goldberg J, Miles TP, et al. Regional variation in the incidence of hip fracture. US white women aged 65 years and older. *JAMA* 1990;264:500–2.

27. Cooper C, Campion G, Melton LJ III. Hip fractures in the elderly: a worldwide projection. *Osteoporos Int* 1992;2:285–9.

28. Royal College of Physicians. Fractured neck of femur – prevention and management. Summary and report of the Royal College of Physicians. *J R Coll Physicians Lond* 1989;23:8–12.

29. Melton LJ III, O'Fallon WM, Riggs BL. Secular trends in the incidence of hip fractures. *Calcif Tissue Int* 1987;41:57–64.

30. Albright F, Smith PH, Richardson AM. Postmenopausal osteoporosis: its clinical features. *JAMA* 1941;116:2465–74.

31. Eastell R, Cedel SL, Wahner HW, et al. Classification of vertebral fractures. *J Bone Miner Res* 1991;6:207–15.

32. Black DM, Cummings SR, Stone K, et al. A new approach to defining normal vertebral dimensions. *J Bone Miner Res* 1991;6:883–92.

33. Cooper C, Atkinson EJ, Jacobsen SJ, et al. Population-based study of survival after osteoporotic fractures. *Am J Epidemiol* 1993;137:1001–5.

34. van Staa TP, Dennison EM, Leufkens HG, et al. Epidemiology of fractures in England and Wales. *Bone* 2001;29:517–22.

35. Melton LJ III, Lane AW, Cooper C, et al. Prevalence and incidence of vertebral deformities. *Osteoporos Int* 1993;3:113–19.

36. O'Neill TW, Felsenberg D, Varlow J, et al. The prevalence of vertebral deformity in European men and women: the European Vertebral Osteoporosis Study. *J Bone Miner Res* 1996;11:1010–18.

37. Ettinger B, Block JE, Smith R, et al. An examination of the association between vertebral deformities, physical disabilities and psychosocial problems. *Maturitas* 1988;10:283–96.

38. Ross PD, Ettinger B, Davis JW, et al. Evaluation of adverse health outcomes associated with vertebral fractures. *Osteoporos Int* 1991;1:134–40.

39. Browner WS, Seeley DG, Vogt TM, et al. Study of Osteoporotic Fractures Research Group. Non-trauma mortality in elderly women with low bone mineral density. *Lancet* 1991;338:355–8.

40. Johansson SJ, Gardsell P, Mellstrom D, et al. Bone mineral measurement is a predictor of survival. *Bone Miner* 1992;17(Suppl 1):166.

41. Oleksik A, Lips P, Dawson A, et al. Health-related quality of life in postmenopausal women with low BMD with or without prevalent vertebral fractures. *J Bone Miner Res* 2000;15:1384–92.

42. Ringe JD. Clinical evaluation of salmon calcitonin in bone pain. In: Christiansen C, Johansen JS, Riggs BJ, eds. *Proceedings of the International Symposium on Osteoporosis*. Volume 2. Copenhagen: Osteoporosis ApS, 1987:1262–4.

43. Kanis JA, McCloskey EV. Epidemiology of vertebral osteoporosis. *Bone* 1992;13:S1–10.

44. Pogrund H, Makin M, Robin G, et al. Osteoporosis in patients with fractured femoral neck in Jerusalem. *Clin Orthop* 1977;124:165–72.

45. Harma M, Heliovaara M, Aromaa A, et al. Thoracic spine compression fractures in Finland. *Clin Orthop* 1986;205:188–94.

46. Smith RW Jr, Rizek J. Epidemiologic studies of osteoporosis in women of Puerto Rico and southeastern Michigan with special reference to age, race, national origin and to other related or associated findings. *Clin Orthop* 1966;45:31–48.

47. Orimo H, Fujiwara S. Epidemiology of vertebral fracture in Asia. *Spine* 1994;8:13–21.

48. Melton LJ III, Atkinson EJ, Cooper C, et al. Vertebral fractures predict subsequent fractures. *Osteoporos Int* 1999;10:214–21.

49. Cooper C, Atkinson EJ, Kotowicz M, et al. Secular trends in the incidence of postmenopausal vertebral fractures. *Calcif Tissue Int* 1992;51:100–4.

50. Bengner U, Johnell O, Redlund-Jonell I. Changes in incidence and prevalence of vertebral fractures during 30 years. *Calcif Tissue Int* 1988;42:293–6.

51. Hansen MA, Overgaard K, Goffredson A, et al. Does the prevalence of vertebral fractures increase? In: Christiansen C, Overgaard K, eds. *Osteoporosis.* Copenhagen: Osteopress ApS, 1990:95.

52. Crawford-Adams J. *Outline of Fractures including joint injuries.* 9th Edition. Edinburgh: Churchill Livingstone, 1987:165.

53. Greendale GA, Barret-Connor E. Outcomes of osteoporotic fractures. In: Marcus R, Feldman D, Kelsey J, eds. *Osteoporosis.* 2nd Edition. San Diego: Academic Press, 2001:819–29.

54. Kaukonen JP, Karaharju EO, Porras M, et al. Functional recovery after fractures of the distal forearm: analysis of radiographic and other factors affecting the outcome. *Ann Chir Gynaecol* 1988;77:27–31.

55. O'Neill TW, Cooper C, Finn JD, et al. Incidence of distal forearm fracture in British men and women. *Osteoporos Int* 2001;12:555–8.

56. Melton LJ III, Cooper C. Magnitude and impact of osteoporosis and fractures. In: Marcus R, Feldman D, Kelsey J, eds: *Osteoporosis.* 2nd Edition (Vol 1). San Diego: Academic Press, 2001:557–67.

57. Department of Health. *Advisory Group on Osteoporosis.* London: Department of Health, 1994.

58. Royal College of Physicians. Osteoporosis: Clinical Guidelines for Prevention and Treatment. London: Royal College of Physicians, 1999.

59. Cooper C. Epidemiology of osteoporosis. *Osteoporos Int* 1999;9(Suppl 2):S2–S8.

60. Praemer A, Furner S, Rice DP. *Musculoskeletal conditions in the United States.* Park Ridge, IL: American Academy of Orthopaedic Surgeons, 1992.

61. van Staa TP, Leufkens HG, Abenhaim L, et al. Use of oral corticosteroids and risk of fractures. *J Bone Miner Res* 2000;15:993–1000.

62. van Staa TP, Leufkens HG, Abenhaim L, et al. Oral corticosteroids and fracture risk: relationship to daily and cumulative doses. *Rheumatology* 2000;39:1383–9.

63. Bone and Tooth Society of Great Britain, National Osteoporosis Society, Royal College of Physicians. *Glucocorticoid-induced osteoporosis: guidelines for prevention and treatment.* London: Royal College of Physicians, 2002. Available at www.rcplondon.ac.uk/pubs/books/glucocorticoid. Accessed June 19, 2004.

2

The Pathogenesis of Osteoporosis

Juliet Compston

Bone composition and structure

The skeleton provides a rigid framework for the body, acting as a site for the attachment of muscles, protecting vital organs, and housing the bone marrow. It contains 99% of total body calcium and phosphate, providing a large reservoir of these ions and playing a major role in the preservation of calcium and phosphate homeostasis. Bone consists of an extracellular collagenous matrix, composed predominantly of type I collagen, proteoglycans, and noncollagenous proteins, including osteocalcin (bone γ-carboxyglutamic acid [GLA] protein), matrix GLA protein, osteonectin, and cell attachment proteins such as fibronectin, osteopontin, thrombospondin, and bone sialoproteins. Bone matrix also contains growth factors that play an important regulatory role in bone modeling and remodeling. These include transforming growth factor (TGF)-βI, -βII, and -βIII, platelet-derived growth factors, insulin-like growth factors (IGFs), epidermal growth factor, and bone morphogenetic proteins. Bone mineral is deposited within the matrix, initially as amorphous calcium phosphate and subsequently mainly in the form of calcium hydroxyapatite.

Cortical or compact bone, which forms approximately 90% of the skeleton, is found mainly in the shafts of long bones and surfaces of flat bones. It is composed of compact bone laid down concentrically around central canals (Haversian systems), which contain blood vessels, lymphatic vessels, nerves, and connective tissue (**Figure 2.1**). Trabecular or cancellous bone is found mainly at the ends of long bones and in the inner parts of flat bones, and consists of interconnecting plates and bars containing hematopoietic or fatty marrow (**Figure 2.2**).

In the adult human skeleton, collagen fibers adopt a preferential orientation, resulting in the formation of lamellar bone. In cancellous bone, the lamellae are arranged parallel to one another, whereas in cortical bone they are concentrically arranged. Woven bone, which is formed in the growing skeleton and in some disease states, is characterized by the random orientation of collagen fibers, and the nonuniform size and distribution of osteocytes.

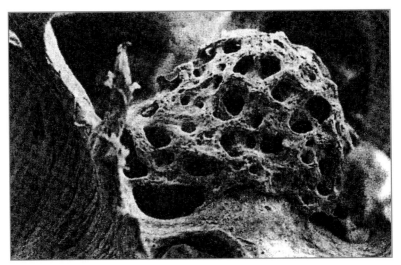

Figure 2.1 Cortical bone from a human iliac crest biopsy showing Haversian canals surrounded by concentric lamellae of compact bone, viewed by polarized light microscopy.

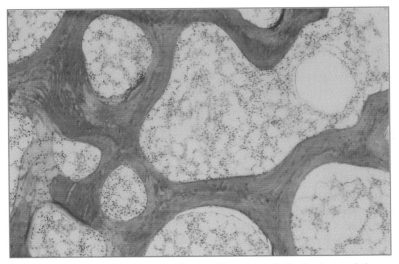

Figure 2.2 Cancellous bone from a human iliac crest biopsy demonstrating the characteristic interconnecting structure.

Bone cells

The three main cell types in bone are osteoblasts, osteoclasts, and osteocytes. However, other cells in the bone microenvironment – including monocytes,

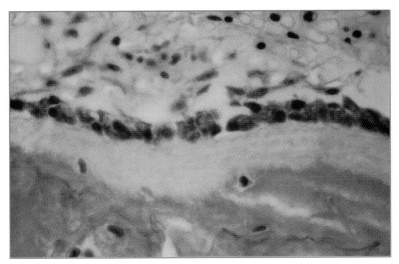

Figure 2.3 An actively forming surface showing osteoblasts on an osteoid seam in human cancellous bone.

lymphocytes, and megakaryocytes – play a vital role in the production of osteogenic cells and the regulation of bone remodeling.

Osteoblasts

Osteoblasts are derived from pluripotent stromal stem cells (**Figure 2.3**) [1]. The factors determining commitment of these cells to a particular lineage (fibroblasts, myoblasts, adipocytes, osteoblasts, or chondrocytes) have not been completely defined, but the transcription factor core binding factor (Cbfa)1 is critical in osteoblast development [2]. Thus, deletion of the gene in mice results in a cartilaginous skeleton lacking bone, and haploinsufficiency in humans is associated with the condition of cleidocranial dysplasia [3]. Regulators of other lineages are also shown in **Figure 2.4**.

Osteoblasts are responsible for the formation and subsequent mineralization of bone matrix; they synthesize growth factors that are secreted and stored within the bone matrix. When actively involved in bone formation, they appear as plump cuboidal cells in close juxtaposition on newly formed osteoid. Some die by the process of apoptosis, while others are buried within mineralized bone to become osteocytes or lining cells (thin flattened cells covering quiescent bone surfaces) (**Figure 2.5**).

Osteoclasts

Osteoclasts are large, multinucleated cells that are derived from hematopoietic precursors of the monocyte–macrophage lineage. They perform the unique function of resorption of mineralized bone (**Figure 2.6**) [4]. They are formed by

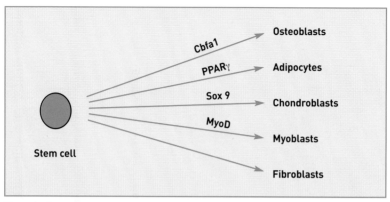

Figure 2.4 Development of osteoblasts and other cell types from stromal stem cells.

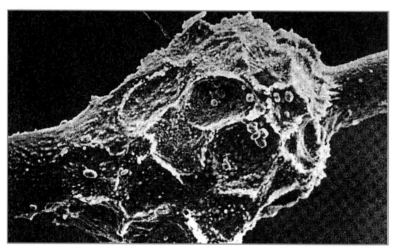

Figure 2.5 Quiescent bone surface showing lining cells on the endosteal membrane covering mineralized bone.

the fusion of mononuclear cells and are characterized by the presence of a ruffled border. During the process of resorption, hydrogen ions generated by carbonic anhydrase II are pumped across the ruffled border by a proton pump to dissolve bone mineral. Lysosomal enzymes, including cysteine proteinases, are then released to degrade the bone matrix (**Figure 2.7**).

Attachment of osteoclasts to mineralized bone is an essential part of the resorption process and is mediated by integrins (adhesion molecules on the cytoplasmic membranes that bind to bone matrix molecules through specific amino-acid sequences) [5]. These attachment proteins include osteopontin,

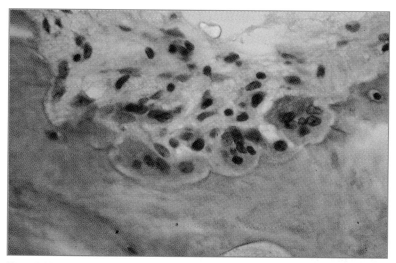

Figure 2.6 Large, multinucleated osteoclasts within a resorption cavity in cancellous iliac crest bone from a patient with Paget's disease.

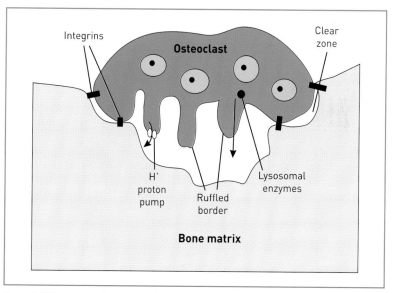

Figure 2.7 The process of bone resorption.

fibronectin, collagen, and bone sialoprotein. Morphologically, attachment of the osteoclast to the bone surface is seen as an actin-containing ring, which completely surrounds the ruffled border [6].

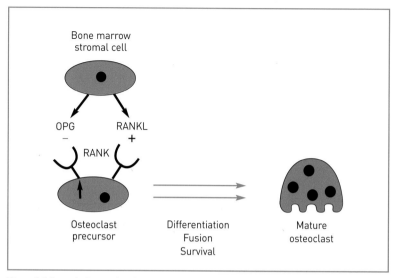

Figure 2.8 Control of osteoclast formation and function: receptor activator of nuclear factor-κB (RANK) ligand and its receptors. OPG: osteoprotegerin.

Many factors are involved in the development of osteoclasts from their hematopoietic precursors. Of particular importance are macrophage colony-stimulating factor (M-CSF) and receptor activator of nuclear factor-κB (RANK) ligand (RANKL), which are produced by osteoblastic cells and are essential for normal osteoclastogenesis [7,8]. The signaling receptor for RANKL is RANK, a type 1 transmembrane protein expressed by osteoclastic cells, whereas osteoprotegerin (OPG) acts as a soluble decoy receptor that prevents RANKL from binding to and activating RANK (**Figure 2.8**) [9].

Apoptosis is an important determinant of osteoclast activity and is regulated by a number of cytokines and hormones [10]. Parathyroid hormone (PTH), 1,25-dihydroxyvitamin D (1,25[OH]$_2$D$_3$), interleukin (IL)-1, IL-6, tumor necrosis factor (TNF)-α, and M-CSF inhibit osteoclast apoptosis, whereas TGF-β acts as a stimulator of apoptosis. RANKL also has antiapoptotic effects, while OPG stimulates osteoclast apoptosis.

Osteocytes

Osteocytes are small, flattened cells within the bone matrix that are connected to one another and to lining cells on the bone surface (**Figure 2.9**). In cortical bone they are arranged circumferentially around the concentric bone lamellae, whereas in cancellous bone they lie parallel to the axis of the collagen fibers. In woven bone, osteocytes are larger and exhibit a more haphazard distribution.

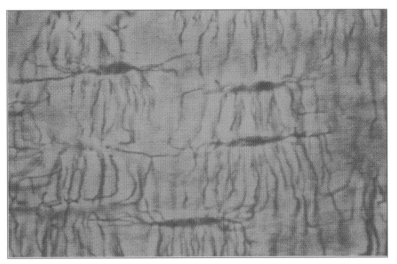

Figure 2.9 Osteocytes in cancellous bone. Note the extensive osteocyte–canalicular network.

Osteocytes are derived from active osteoblasts and play an important role in the osteogenic response to mechanical stimuli, 'sensing' physical strains and initiating an appropriate modeling or remodeling response via the production of a cascade of chemical messengers, including glucose-6-dehydrogenase, nitric oxide, and IGFs [11]. The life span of osteocytes is critically dependent on and inversely related to bone turnover; thus, in high bone turnover states, osteocytes are liberated by the process of bone resorption. Osteocytes are terminally differentiated cells and ultimately undergo apoptosis or are phagocytosed by osteoclasts during bone resorption.

Bone remodeling

Bone remodeling occurs in both cortical and cancellous bone and is a process by which old bone is removed and subsequently replaced by new bone [12]. It occurs at discrete sites on the bone surface, termed bone remodeling units, and is the process whereby a quantum of mineralized bone is removed by osteoclasts, followed by the synthesis and mineralization of osteoid by osteoblasts within the created cavity (**Figure 2.10**).

After resorption has been completed, there is a short reversal phase in which a highly mineralized, collagen-poor cement line is laid down at the base of the cavity. Local factors released from the bone matrix during the resorptive phase might be responsible for the chemotactic attraction of osteoblast precursors to the remodeling site, while growth factors released by nearby osteoblasts are believed to stimulate the proliferation and differentiation of these cells.

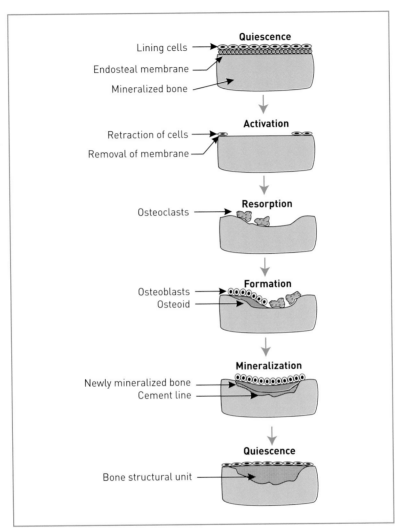

Figure 2.10 The process of bone remodeling.

Under normal circumstances, the temporal sequence is always that of resorption followed by formation (coupling), and the amounts of bone resorbed and formed within individual remodeling units are quantitatively similar (balance). The newly formed bone, which represents the end stage of the remodeling process, is known as a bone structural unit. The time taken for completion of a bone structural unit in the adult human skeleton is approximately 3–6 months, most of which is occupied by the formative phase [13].

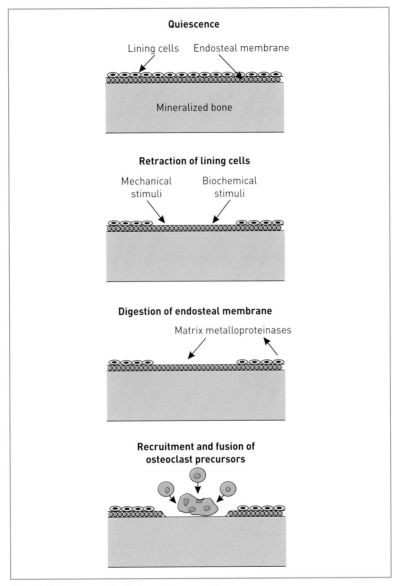

Figure 2.11 The process of activation of bone remodeling.

Activation is the process by which the quiescent bone surface is prepared for resorption. It involves retraction of the lining cells and removal of the thin collagenous membrane covering the mineralized bone surface (**Figure 2.11**).

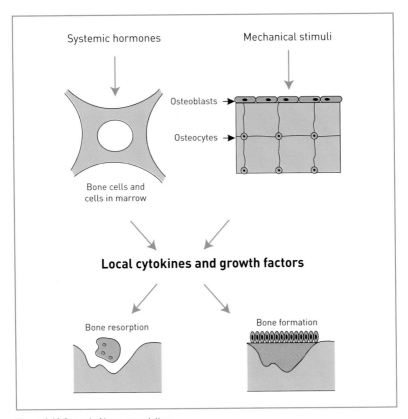

Figure 2.12 Control of bone remodeling.

The mechanisms responsible for activation of bone remodeling are poorly understood, but there is evidence that matrix metalloproteinases, produced by osteoblasts, are involved in the latter process. The spatial distribution of bone remodeling units is unlikely to be random, and site-specific activation may be achieved by mechanical stresses transmitted to the lining cells via the osteocytic–canalicular network.

Control of bone remodeling

The control of bone remodeling is complex and results from the interaction of mechanical stresses, systemic hormones, and locally produced cytokines, prostaglandins, and growth factors (**Figure 2.12**). The latter, produced by bone cells or cells in the bone microenvironment, act in an autocrine or paracrine manner and are likely to mediate, at least in part, the effects of mechanical stimuli and systemic hormones. In addition to these factors, other mechanisms and mediators are also involved in the regulation of bone remodeling. These include prostacyclins, nitric oxide, oxygen-derived free radicals, constitutively

Agent	Abbreviation
Stimulators of bone resorption	
Interleukin-1, -6, -8, -11	IL-1, -6, -8, -11
Tumor necrosis factor	TNF
Epidermal growth factor	EGF
Platelet-derived growth factor	PDGF
Fibroblast growth factor	FGF
Leukemia inhibitory factor	LIF
Macrophage colony-stimulating factor	M-CSF
Granulocyte/macrophage colony-stimulating factor	GM-CSF
Inhibitors of bone resorption	
Interferon-γ	IFN-γ
Interleukin-4	IL-4
Stimulators of bone formation	
Insulin-like growth factor	IGF
Transforming growth factor-β	TGF-β
Fibroblast growth factor	FGF
Platelet-derived growth factor	PDGF
Bone morphogenetic protein	BMP

Table 2.1 Cytokines and growth factors that affect bone.

produced receptor antagonists (eg, IL-1 receptor antagonist) and cell–cell contact. A large number of cytokines and growth factors have been shown to affect bone cells *in vitro* and, in some cases, *in vivo*. Many of these have multiple actions on both osteoblasts and osteoclasts and act interdependently with other factors [14]. Their main effects are shown in **Table 2.1**.

IL-1 and TNFs are potent stimulators of bone resorption and have been implicated in the osteolysis associated with myeloma, and the juxta-articular osteoporosis associated with rheumatoid arthritis. M-CSF is essential for the formation of osteoclasts, and its absence in mice results in the development of osteopetrosis. The TGFs and fibroblast growth factors are powerful stimulators of bone formation: the bone morphogenetic proteins, which are members of the TGF superfamily, possess the unique property of stimulating *de novo* bone formation in a manner analogous to fracture repair and endochondral ossification.

Mechanical stimuli are a major determinant of the size, shape, and microarchitecture of bones during skeletal growth, and they subsequently play an important role in the maintenance of bone mass.

Hormones

Many systemic hormones influence bone modeling during growth and bone remodeling in adult life. These include PTH, tri-iodothyronine, growth hormone, glucocorticoids, $1,25(OH)_2D_3$, and the sex steroids [15]. The effects of PTH depend on its mode of administration and, possibly, dose. Thus, continuous administration results in increased bone turnover, particularly in cortical bone, resulting in bone loss, whereas intermittent administration produces an anabolic effect. Bone resorption is stimulated by $1,25(OH)_2D_3$ *in vitro*, probably via effects on the differentiation of osteoclast precursors and their subsequent fusion to form mature osteoclasts. It also stimulates the synthesis of osteocalcin and alkaline phosphatase by osteoblasts.

In patients with rickets or osteomalacia, $1,25(OH)_2D_3$ promotes the mineralization of bone, an effect mediated by increased circulating calcium and phosphate concentrations. Growth hormone plays an important role in skeletal growth, increasing bone turnover with a net increase in bone mass, and in periosteal apposition of bone – effects that are mediated, at least in part, by IGFs.Tri-iodothyronine also increases bone turnover, with a net decrease in bone mass in both cortical and cancellous bone. Finally, calcitonin is one of very few factors known to affect osteoclasts directly, causing inhibition of osteoclastic resorption by effects on both precursor and mature cells.

Estrogen and testosterone

The effects of estrogen on bone are mediated through both genomic and nongenomic effects. Two main subtypes of estrogen receptor (ER) have been described, ER-α and ER-β, each of which has several isoforms [16]. The tissue distribution of the two main subtypes is overlapping but not identical, and their respective functions remain to be fully defined. ERs are present on osteoblasts, osteoclasts, and osteocytes; in addition, they are present on mononuclear cells and megakaryocytes in the bone marrow [17].

The bone-preserving effects of estrogen are mediated predominantly through effects on osteoclast number and activity that, in turn, result from the reduced production of proresorptive cytokines (eg, IL-1, IL-6, TNF-α, RANKL, and granulocyte M-CSF) by bone cells and cells in the bone microenvironment [18]. Estrogen also increases the production of IL-1 receptor antagonist, TGF-β, and OPG – in combination, these changes result in reduced generation of osteoclasts and increased osteoclast apoptosis. High doses of estrogen have been shown to increase bone formation, both in animals and in humans [19,20]. The mechanisms by which this is mediated are incompletely understood, but may involve increased production of TGF-β, IGFs, and platelet-derived growth factors.

Testosterone also has an effect on bone, mediated via the androgen receptor. However, estrogens are also believed to play an important role in skeletal homeostasis in males and can be formed from androgens in the bone

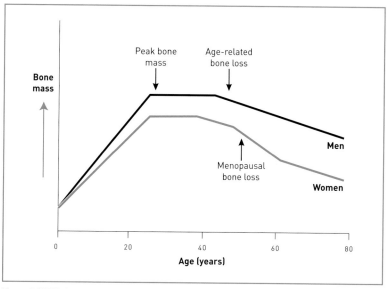

Figure 2.13 Lifetime changes in bone mass.

microenvironment by the enzyme aromatase. The importance of estrogens in the male skeleton is illustrated by the failure of normal bone development in a male with ER resistance but normal circulating testosterone levels [21] and the significant relationship between bone mineral density (BMD) and serum estradiol, but not serum testosterone, in healthy older men [22].

Glucocorticoids

Glucocorticoids have complex effects on bone, but the predominant effect is a reduction in bone formation resulting from the inhibition of osteoblast generation and activity; the latter resulting from increased osteoblast apoptosis [23,24]. Glucocorticoids may also increase bone resorption by increasing osteoclastogenesis and reducing osteoclast apoptosis [25]. This effect is most evident in the early stages of glucocorticoid therapy, and may account for the more rapid rates of bone loss and fracture in the first few months of treatment.

The mechanisms responsible for these effects have not been fully defined, but include an increase in the production of RANKL and a decrease in the production of OPG. Hypogonadism also contributes to glucocorticoid-induced bone loss, as does reduced intestinal calcium absorption and increased renal calcium excretion. The role of secondary hyperparathyroidism in glucocorticoid-induced bone loss is, however, controversial.

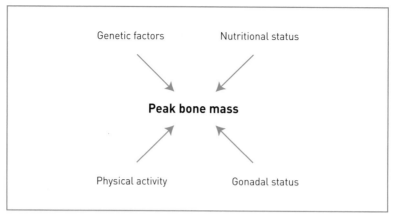

Figure 2.14 Determinants of peak bone mass.

Lifetime changes in bone mass

During childhood and adolescence there is rapid linear and appositional skeletal growth, the former reaching a maximum in the latter half of the second decade of life. Bone mass then continues to increase by appositional growth, and peak bone mass is attained during the third decade of life. Age-related bone loss probably commences during the fourth decade and continues throughout life, accelerating in women during the years around the menopause (**Figure 2.13**). The rate and onset of bone loss varies according to the skeletal site and, because of its large surface-to-volume ratio and greater potential for metabolic activity, losses in cancellous bone exceed those in cortical bone. Overall, it is estimated that approximately 50% of cancellous and 35% of cortical bone mass are lost over a lifetime in women, with losses in men approximately two-thirds of these amounts.

Peak bone mass

The peak bone mass attained is a major determinant of subsequent bone mass and fracture risk in later life. When expressed in terms of areal bone density, which corrects only partially for bone size, peak bone mass is greater in men than in women, although these differences are reduced or even reversed if bone mass is expressed as volumetric bone density. Marked racial differences in peak bone mass also occur, with higher values in American blacks than in Caucasians, and the lowest values in Asians and the Japanese. The factors determining peak bone mass are only partially understood (**Figure 2.14**). Genetic influences are clearly important, as demonstrated by racial differences in bone mass and the greater concordance of bone mass in monozygotic as opposed to dizygotic twins. Some of this effect is likely to be mediated via skeletal size, but there is also evidence that polymorphisms in the vitamin D receptor gene and other genes may influence bone mass [26].

Other factors that influence peak bone mass are nutrition (particularly dietary calcium intake), physical activity, and gonadal status. Since the transverse diameter of bones continues to increase throughout life because of periosteal appositional growth, the rate of bone loss in later life is likely to be underestimated when assessed by techniques that measure areal or linear BMD. In addition, cross-sectional studies are subject to survivor bias and are often unrepresentative of the general population because of the exclusion of subjects with fractures. These factors also result in underestimation of rates of bone loss. Finally, the accuracy of measurements in the spine decreases with age because of the increased prevalence of osteophytes, extraskeletal calcification, and vertebral deformity, all of which will produce artifactually high values for BMD, and hence underestimate bone loss.

Pathophysiology of bone loss

At the cellular level, two basic mechanisms of bone loss exist. Quantitatively, the most important of these is an increase in activation frequency (increased bone turnover), the effect of which is to increase the number of remodeling units on the bone surface that are undergoing resorption at any given time. The area occupied by resorption cavities is known as the remodeling space, and administration of an agent that reduces activation frequency leads to a small initial gain in bone mass due to infilling of these cavities.

The other mechanism of bone loss, which may operate independently or in conjunction with increased activation frequency, is remodeling imbalance, in which the amount of bone formed within individual bone remodeling units is less than that resorbed due to an increase in erosion depth and/or a reduction in the amount formed. This form of bone loss is irreversible within that remodeling unit once the remodeling cycle has been completed.

Postmenopausal bone loss

Menopausal bone loss is associated with both increased activation frequency and remodeling imbalance (**Figure 2.15**) [8]. The former appears to be a direct consequence of estrogen deficiency, showing a close temporal relationship with estrogen withdrawal and responding rapidly to estrogen repletion. The negative remodeling balance, which is a feature of age-related bone loss in both men and women, is less clearly related to estrogen status, although there is some evidence that it can be corrected by estrogen replacement.

Histomorphometric data in women with postmenopausal osteoporosis show evidence of striking heterogeneity in the indices of bone turnover, with low, normal, and high values all represented. Several factors are likely to contribute to the wide range of changes observed, including measurement variance, skeletal heterogeneity, intermittency of changes in bone turnover, and differences in patient selection. Furthermore, changes in bone turnover after the menopause may be sequential, with high turnover in the early stages of

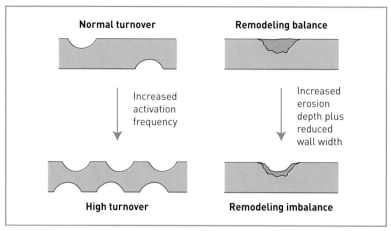

Figure 2.15 Cellular mechanisms of menopausal bone loss.

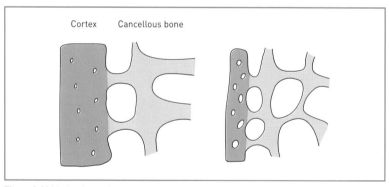

Figure 2.16 Mechanisms of cortical bone loss, showing trabecularization of endocortical surface and increased cortical porosity.

the menopause decreasing in later years. A much more consistent finding in these patients is that of a decreased wall width when compared with age- and sex-matched control subjects, indicating reduced bone formation at the cellular level. Whether this reflects a specific osteoblast defect in postmenopausal osteoporosis is uncertain. An alternative explanation could be that smaller bone structural units are associated with a lower peak bone mass, and thus a predisposition to osteoporosis.

The changes in erosion depth associated with estrogen deficiency have not been clearly established. The rapid evolution of structural disruption of cancellous bone architecture associated with estrogen deficiency suggests that increased osteoclastic activity, resulting in trabecular penetration, is likely to occur in the early stages of estrogen deficiency. However, direct evidence to support this

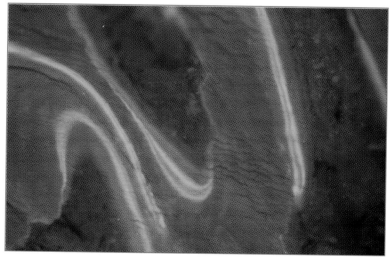

Figure 2.17 Double tetracycline labeling in bone, viewed by fluorescence microscopy.

hypothesis is, at present, lacking in humans; measurements of erosion depth in women with postmenopausal osteoporosis have generally revealed values close to normal. This might reflect the early and transient nature of osteoclastic trabecular penetration associated with estrogen deficiency and the inability to measure resorption cavities that have caused this change.

Age-related cortical bone loss

Age-related cortical bone loss occurs by two mechanisms: endosteal bone resorption and increased cortical porosity resulting from a negative remodeling imbalance (**Figure 2.16**). The former exceeds periosteal appositional growth, resulting in a reduction in cortical width as aging progresses.

Histomorphometric assessment of bone remodeling

Bone histomorphometry is an important research tool in the investigation of pathophysiologic changes in osteoporosis and the mechanisms by which therapeutic interventions affect bone mass and structure. Using histologic sections obtained from iliac crest biopsies, a detailed quantitative assessment of bone remodeling and architecture can be obtained *in vivo*, providing information that cannot be gained from other investigations such as bone densitometry or the measurement of biochemical indices of bone turnover.

Bone turnover

Bone turnover is assessed using the technique of double tetracycline labeling, in which the patient is given two time-spaced doses of oral tetracycline prior to biopsy. Tetracycline binds to mineralizing surfaces and can be visualized by

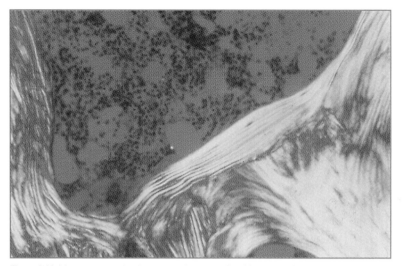

Figure 2.18 A bone structural unit, representing a completed bone remodeling unit, viewed by polarized light microscopy. The boundaries are formed by the cement line and mineralized bone surface.

fluorescence microscopy (**Figure 2.17**). Its surface extent provides an indication of the actively forming surface, while the separation of the two labels is used to calculate the mineral appositional rate [27]. From these primary measurements, the bone formation rate at tissue level can be calculated, providing an index of bone turnover.

Resorption rates and activation frequency
No equivalent marker exists for the assessment of bone surface currently undergoing either activation or resorption [28]. Resorption rates and activation frequency can therefore only be indirectly assessed from bone formation rates, based on the assumptions that bone resorption and formation are coupled in time and space, and that a steady state exists with respect to bone remodeling – neither of which is likely to be tenable in many cases of untreated or treated osteoporosis. Accurate data on resorption rates and activation frequency must therefore await the development of markers of activation and resorption, analogous to tetracycline labeling for the assessment of bone formation.

Remodeling balance
Remodeling balance can be assessed by measurements of the amount of bone resorbed and formed within individual bone remodeling units. The amount of bone formed is represented by the mean wall width, a measurement performed on completed bone structural units (**Figure 2.18**), which can be most easily visualized by polarized light microscopy. In some situations, it will be desirable to distinguish between newly formed structural units and those that have

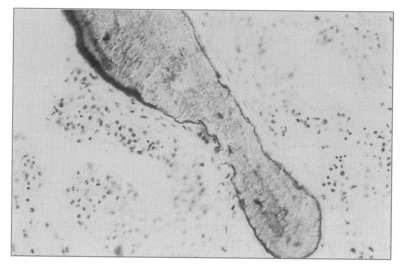

Figure 2.19 Resorption cavity in human iliac crest cancellous bone, containing resorbing cells. Note the adjacent osteoid, indicating a forming surface.

been present for longer periods of time. This can be achieved by paired measurements of osteoid thickness and wall thickness in structural units that have not yet been completed.

Resorption depth

The assessment of resorption depth is more problematic due to difficulties associated with the identification of resorption cavities and the definition of those cells in which resorption has been completed. The use of polarized light microscopy to demonstrate the interruption of lamellae at the edges of the cavity, and resorbing cells within the cavity, assists identification. However, artifacts formed during the production of bone sections may result in errors of identification, and the absence of resorbing cells within a cavity in histologic sections does not exclude the presence of active resorption (**Figure 2.19**).

Resorption cavities

The identification of cavities in which resorption has been completed can only be made with certainty when a thin layer of osteoid is present at the base of the cavity, indicating that the formative phase has commenced. Two direct approaches to the quantitative assessment of resorption cavities have been described. In the first, the number of lamellae eroded beneath the bone surface is counted and the resorptive site is reconstructed using identification of different cell types associated with different stages of completion of the resorption process (osteoclastic, mononuclear, and preosteoblastic) [13]. Although in theory this method enables the measurement of final resorption depth, the identification of different cell types on morphologic grounds is difficult and prone to inaccuracy.

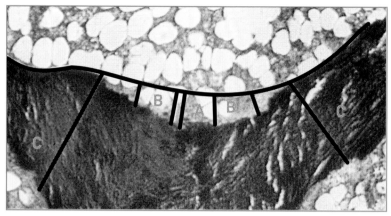

Figure 2.20 Reconstruction of the eroded bone surface using a computer-generated cubic spline. Four lines **(B)** are used to measure the mean erosion depth; **A** represents the maximum depth, and **C** the trabecular width on either side of the cavity. Reproduced with permission from Elsevier [29].

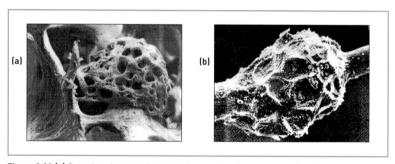

Figure 2.21 (a) Scanning electron microscope image of a 1.5-mm microcallus formation. **(b)** Microcallus formation with clearly recognizable resorption on the surface. Reproduced from *J Bone Miner Res* 1995;10:1410–16 with permission of the American Society for Bone and Mineral Research [31].

The other approach involves reconstruction of the eroded bone surface [29], which may be computer-assisted or manual (**Figure 2.20**). This method does not differentiate between cavities at different stages of completion, providing an assessment of the mean depth of all cavities present, and thus underestimates the completed resorption depth.

Structural mechanisms of bone loss

The alterations in bone remodeling associated with age-related bone loss and osteoporosis determine the accompanying changes in bone architecture, an important determinant of bone strength and fracture risk [30]. Both cortical and cancellous bone make important contributions to the mechanical properties of the skeleton – the former by virtue of its compact nature and the latter by its interconnectedness and the preferential orientation of trabeculae, which develop in response to mechanical stresses during skeletal development. Other determinants of bone strength include bone mass, geometry, composition, and the balance between fatigue microdamage and its repair (**Figure 2.21**) [31].

In cancellous bone, bone loss may be accompanied by trabecular thinning or trabecular penetration and erosion (**Figure 2.22**). These two mechanisms are, to some extent, interdependent and commonly coexist [32]. Trabecular thinning is associated with a better preservation of bone architecture than penetration and erosion, although, as the trabeculae become progressively thinner, the likelihood of penetration increases. Trabecular penetration and erosion result in greater structural disruption for a given reduction in bone mass than trabecular thinning; the accompanying reduction in connectivity also produces proportionately greater adverse mechanical effects. Furthermore, whereas trabecular thickening in response to therapeutic agents is well documented, it remains unlikely that bone structure, once disrupted by trabecular penetration and erosion, can be fully restored.

Low bone-turnover states (eg, osteoporosis associated with long-term glucocorticoid therapy and chronic liver disease) predispose to trabecular thinning, whereas increased erosion depth and/or increased bone turnover will favor trabecular penetration and erosion (changes that are characteristic of bone loss associated with estrogen deficiency) (**Figure 2.23**). Age-related bone loss is accompanied by some degree of trabecular thinning in both sexes. However, while this mechanism predominates in men, trabecular penetration and erosion constitute the major structural change in postmenopausal women [33].

Assessment of cancellous bone structure

The mechanical properties of cancellous bone are dependent upon a number of aspects of its structure; these include trabecular size and spacing, connectivity, and anisotropy. Trabecular width and spacing can be measured directly or calculated using area and perimeter measurements. The latter approach assumes a parallel plate model, which may not be valid for osteoporotic bone.

Connectivity is a three-dimensional quality that describes the presence of multiple junctions between nodes or junctions and can only be measured directly on three-dimensional images. However, using two-dimensional images, other methods have been described that provide indirect information about

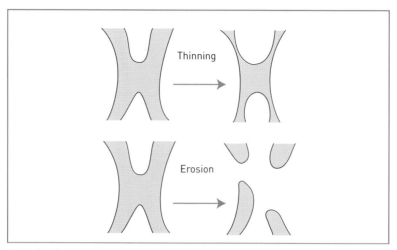

Figure 2.22 Structural mechanisms of cancellous bone loss.

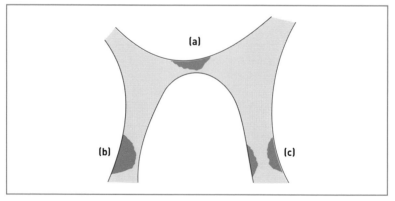

Figure 2.23 Mechanisms of trabecular penetration. **(a)** Trabecular thinning and normal resorption cavity. **(b)** Increased osteoclastic activity resulting in increased erosion depth. **(c)** Increased activation frequency leading to greater likelihood of two resorption cavities at opposite sides on a trabecula.

connectivity and other aspects of bone structure. These include strut analysis (**Figure 2.24**), marrow star volume, and trabecular bone pattern factor [34].

Anisotropy describes deviation from a preferred orientation of a structure and is likely to be an important determinant of mechanical strength. Its quantitative assessment provides a particularly difficult challenge, but measurement in three-dimensional images of bone has been described.

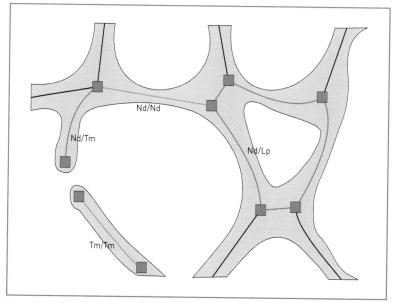

Figure 2.24 Strut analysis, illustrating node-to-node (Nd/Nd), node-to-loop (Nd/Lp), node-to-terminus (Nd/Tm), and terminus-to-terminus (Tm/Tm) strut types. Structural integrity is positively related to the Nd/Tm ratio and the Nd/Nd and Nd/Lp strut lengths, and inversely related to Nd/Tm and Tm/Tm strut lengths.

Effects of drugs on bone remodeling and structure

Although changes in BMD in response to drugs used in the treatment of osteoporosis have been widely documented, relatively little information exists about the effects of these drugs on bone remodeling and structure. In particular, the cellular mechanisms by which increases in bone mass are mediated in response to anabolic drugs, such as sodium fluoride and PTH, have not been clearly established, and information on drug-induced effects on bone structure is sparse.

Suppression of bone turnover

Drugs that act predominantly by suppression of bone turnover include estrogens, androgens, bisphosphonates, calcitonin, and vitamin D. However, the differential effects of these drugs on the processes of activation and resorption have not been clearly defined. The magnitude of the therapeutic effect will depend on both the pretreatment level of bone turnover and the degree of suppression achieved.

In theory, therefore, patients with low turnover osteoporosis will show little or no response to antiresorptive agents, whereas those with high turnover osteoporosis will be the most responsive. This hypothesis remains to be formally

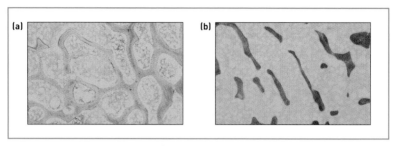

Figure 2.25 Iliac crest cancellous bone **(a)** before and **(b)** 6 months after the induction of estrogen deficiency by gonadotropin-releasing hormone analog therapy in a 28-year-old woman with endometriosis. Reproduced with permission from Elsevier [35].

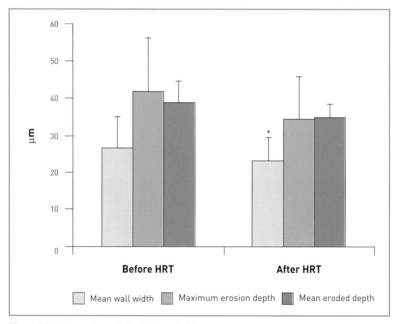

Figure 2.26 Indices of remodeling balance in 22 postmenopausal women before and after long-term hormone replacement therapy (HRT). Mean duration of therapy 24 months. There is a small, statistically significant reduction in mean wall width and a quantitatively similar, but nonsignificant, decrease in maximum and mean erosion depth. *$p<0.03$.

tested but, if it is correct, provides a rationale for treatment selection based on pretreatment levels of bone turnover. However, spontaneous fluctuations in bone turnover and poor sensitivity of biochemical markers in reflecting regional changes may limit the value of such an approach.

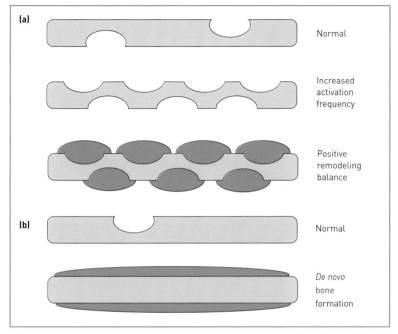

Figure 2.27 Mechanisms of cancellous bone gain in response to anabolic agents. A positive remodeling balance will result in increased cancellous bone volume and trabecular thickening, whether or not activation frequency is increased. **(a)** The combination of positive remodeling balance and increased activation frequency. **(b)** *De novo* bone formation on quiescent bone surfaces represents another mechanism of bone gain. Reproduced with permission from Humana Press [36].

Improvements in remodeling balance

Unlike changes in bone turnover, alterations in remodeling balance are not reflected by biochemical markers and can only be assessed using histomorphometric techniques. Improvements in remodeling balance may be achieved by a reduction in erosion depth and/or an increase in wall width. Measurement of both components is essential, since the impact of a change in one is dependent on the direction and magnitude of change in the other. For example, a reduction in erosion depth will not alter remodeling balance if there is a quantitatively similar reduction in wall width, but it will lead to an improvement if the reduction in wall width is smaller than that in erosion depth.

For drugs that predominantly act by reducing bone turnover, changes in remodeling balance are likely to have only modest effects on bone mass in view of the relatively low number of remodeling units present on the bone surface at any given time. In contrast to the relatively small contribution of drug-induced changes in remodeling balance, their impact on cancellous bone structure may be substantial, with bone loss associated with trabecular penetration and erosion

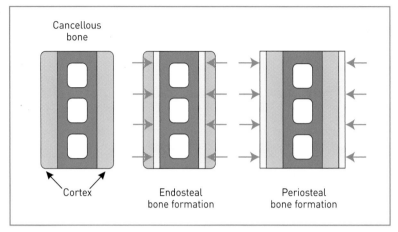

Figure 2.28 Potential effects of anabolic agents on cortical width and bone size. Endosteal new bone formation increases cortical width but not bone diameter, whereas periosteal new bone formation increases both cortical width and the bone diameter. Reproduced with permission from Humana Press [36].

(a reduction in erosion depth should prevent or reduce architectural deterioration) (**Figure 2.25**). In view of the rapid evolution of structural disruption in postmenopausal bone loss, and the likelihood that an early increase in erosion depth is largely responsible for such changes, the effects of estrogen replacement on resorption depth are of particular interest.

Effects of estrogen therapy

Histomorphometric data on the effects of estrogen therapy in postmenopausal women are sparse and limited to relatively long-term studies. These have indicated a small reduction in erosion depth after 1–2 years of treatment (**Figure 2.26**), but the short-term effects are unknown. However, the preservation of bone structure by estrogen replacement therapy would be consistent with a quantitatively greater effect in the early stages of bone loss – a contention also supported by the apparent protection by tibolone against the loss of cancellous bone structure induced by gonadotropin-releasing hormone analogs [35].

Anabolic effects

Mechanisms by which anabolic effects may be achieved in cancellous bone are illustrated in **Figure 2.27** [36]. Firstly, a positive remodeling balance resulting from increased bone formation will produce anabolic effects. If combined with an increase in activation frequency, this has the potential to produce relatively large increases in bone mass. Secondly, *de novo* bone formation, in which new bone is formed either on quiescent bone surfaces in the absence of prior resorption or in the marrow cavity without a pre-existing template of bone, will also increase bone mass and might additionally increase the connectivity of cancellous bone. In the case of intermittent PTH peptide administration, there is evidence that both of these mechanisms contribute to the observed increase in bone mass [37,38].

Potential mechanisms for anabolic effects on cortical bone are illustrated in **Figure 2.28**. An increase in cortical width may result from increased formation at either the endosteal or periosteal surface. The latter, which has been reported in individuals treated with intermittent PTH peptide, increases the external diameter of bone, an important and independent determinant of bone strength.

Effects on cortical porosity might also occur with respect to the number, size, and distribution of canals. Increased cortical porosity has been reported with intermittent PTH peptide treatment, but potential adverse effects on bone strength appear to be outweighed by the increase in cortical width and bone size.

Changes in bone mineralization

After the bone remodeling cycle has been completed, mineralization of the new bone continues (secondary mineralization). The degree of secondary mineralization is inversely related to bone turnover; the lower the bone turnover, the smaller the chance that mineralization will be halted by the process of activation of a new bone remodeling unit at that site. Thus, administration of potent antiresorptive agents (eg, the bisphosphonate alendronate) is associated with increased secondary mineralization, resulting in an increase in the degree of mineralization of bone [39]. This contributes to the sustained increase in BMD observed after treatment with this agent and probably also has beneficial effects on bone strength, although these may be compromised in the long term by increased microdamage resulting from suppression of bone turnover.

References

1. Owen M. Lineage of osteogenic cells and their relationship to the stromal system. In: Peck WA, ed. *Bone and Mineral Research*. New York, NY: Elsevier, 1985:1–26.

2. Komori T, Yagi H, Nomura S, et al. Targeted disruption of Cbfa1 results in a complete lack of bone formation owing to maturational arrest of osteoblasts. *Cell* 1997;89:755–64.

3. Otto F, Thornell AP, Crompton T, et al. Cbfa1, a candidate gene for cleidocranial dysplasia syndrome, is essential for osteoblast differentiation and bone development. *Cell* 1997;89:765–71.

4. Suda T, Nakamura I, Jimi E, et al. Regulation of osteoclast function. *J Bone Miner Res* 1997;12:869–79.

5. Horton MA, Dorey EL, Nesbitt SA, et al. Modulation of vitronectin receptor-mediated osteoclast adhesion by Arg-Gly-Asp peptide analogs: a structure–function analysis. *J Bone Miner Res* 1993;8:239–47.

6. Lakkakorpi PT, Vaananen HK. Cytoskeletal changes in osteoclasts during the resorption cycle. *Microsc Res Technique* 1996;33:171–81.

7. Yoshida H, Hayashi S, Kunisada T, et al. The murine mutation osteopetrosis is in the coding region of the macrophage colony stimulating factor gene. *Nature* 1990;345:442–4.

8. Yasuda H, Shima N, Nakagawa N, et al. Osteoclast differentiation factor is a ligand for osteoprotegerin/ osteoclastogenesis inhibitory factor and is identical to TRANCE/RANKL. *Proc Natl Acad Sci USA* 1998;95:3597–602.

9. Kong YY, Yoshida H, Sarosi I, et al. OPGL is a key regulator of osteoclastogenesis, lymphocyte development and lymph-node organogenesis. *Nature* 1999;397:315–23.

10. Manolagas SC. Birth and death of bone cells: basic regulatory mechanisms and implications for the pathogenesis and treatment of osteoporosis. *Endocr Rev* 2000;21:115–37.

11. Aarden EM, Burger EH, Nijweide PJ. Function of osteocytes in bone. *J Cell Biochem* 1994;55:287–99.

12. Parfitt AM. The cellular basis of bone remodeling. The quantum concept re-examined in light of recent advances in the cell biology of bone. *Calcif Tissue Int* 1984;36:S37–45.

13. Eriksen EF. Normal and pathological remodeling of human trabecular bone: three-dimensional reconstruction of the remodeling sequence in normals and in metabolic bone disease. *Endocr Rev* 1986;7:379–408.

14. Manolagas SC, Jilka RL. Bone marrow, cytokines, and bone remodeling – emerging insights into the pathophysiology of osteoporosis. *N Engl J Med* 1995;332:305–11.

15. Compston JE. Sex steroids and bone. *Physiol Rev* 2001;81:419–47.

16. Kuiper GG, van den Bemd GJ, van Leeuwen JP. Estrogen receptor and the SERM concept. *J Endocrinol Invest* 1999;22:594–603.

17. Bord S, Horner A, Beavan S, et al. Estrogen receptors (ER) α and β are differentially expressed in growing human bone. *J Clin Endocrinol Metab* 2001;86:2309–14.

18. Pacifici R, Brown C, Puscheck E, et al. Effect of surgical menopause and estrogen replacement on cytokine release from human blood mononuclear cells. *Proc Natl Acad Sci USA* 1991;88:5134–8.

19. Edwards MW, Bain SD, Bailey MC, et al. 17β estradiol stimulation of endosteal bone formation in the ovariectomised mouse: an animal model for the evaluation of bone-targeted estrogens. *Bone* 1992;13:29–34.

20. Vedi S, Purdie DW, Ballard P, et al. Bone remodeling and structure in postmenopausal women treated with long-term, high-dose estrogen therapy. *Osteoporos Int* 1999;10:52–8.

21. Smith E, Boyd J, Frank GR, et al. Estrogen resistance caused by a mutation in the estrogen-receptor gene in a man. *N Engl J Med* 1994;331:1056–61.

22. Khosla S, Melton LJ III, Atkinson EJ, et al. Relationship of serum sex steroid levels to longitudinal changes in bone density in young versus elderly men. *Clin Endocrinol Metab* 2001;86:3555–61.

23. Weinstein RS, Nicholas RW, Manolagas SC. Apoptosis of osteocytes in glucocorticoid-induced osteonecrosis of the hip. *J Clin Endocrinol Metab* 2000;85:2907–12.

24. Weinstein RS, Jilka RL, Parfitt AM, Manolagas SC. Inhibition of osteoblastogenesis and promotion of apoptosis of osteoblasts and osteocytes by glucocorticoids – potential mechanisms of their deleterious effects on bone. *J Clin Invest* 1998;102:274–82.

25. Weinstein RS, Chen JR, Powers CC, et al. Promotion of osteoclast survival and antagonism of bisphosphonate-induced osteoclast apoptosis by glucocorticoids. *J Clin Invest* 2002;109:1041–8.

26. Morrison NA, Qi JC, Tokita A, et al. Prediction of bone density from vitamin D receptor alleles. *Nature* 1994;367:284–7.

27. Frost HM. Tetracycline-based histological analysis of bone remodeling. *Calcif Tissue Res* 1969;3:211–37.

28. Compston JE, Croucher PI. Histomorphometric assessment of trabecular bone remodeling in osteoporosis. *Bone Miner* 1991;14:91–102.

29. Garrahan NJ, Croucher PI, Compston JE. A computerized technique for the quantitative assessment of resorption cavities in trabecular bone. *Bone* 1990;11:241–5.

30. Parfitt AM. Implications of architecture for the pathogenesis and prevention of vertebral fracture. *Bone* 1992;13:S41–7.

31. Hahn M, Vogel M, Amling M, et al. Microcallus formations of the cancellous bone: a quantitative analysis of the human spine. *J Bone Miner Res* 1995;10:1410–16.

32. Compston JE, Mellish RW, Croucher P, et al. Structural mechanisms of trabecular bone loss in man. *Bone Miner* 1989;6:339–50.

33. Mellish RW, Garrahan NJ, Compston JE. Age related changes in trabecular width and spacing in human iliac crest biopsies. *Bone Miner* 1989;6:331–8.

34. Compston JE. Connectivity of cancellous bone: assessment and mechanical implications. *Bone* 1994;15:463–6.

35. Compston JE, Yamaguchi K, Croucher PI, et al. The effects of gonadotrophin-releasing hormone agonists on iliac crest cancellous bone structure in women with endometriosis. *Bone* 1995;16:261–7.

36. Compston JE. Mechanisms of bone loss and bone gain in untreated and treated osteoporosis. *Endocrine* 2002;17:21–27.

37. Dempster DW, Cosman F, Kurland ES, et al. Effects of daily treatment with parathyroid hormone on bone microarchitecture and turnover in patients with osteoporosis: a paired biopsy study. *J Bone Miner Res* 2001;16:1846–53.

38. Dempster DW, Cosman F, Kurland ES, et al. Effects of daily treatment with parathyroid hormone on bone microarchitecture and turnover in patients with osteoporosis: a paired biopsy study. *J Bone Miner Res* 2001;16:S179.

39. Boivin G, Chavassieux PM, Santora AC, et al. Alendronate increases bone strength by increasing the mean degree of mineralization of bone tissue in osteoporotic women. *Bone* 2000;27:687–94.

3

Risk Factors for Fracture

Nigel Arden

Introduction

The most important clinical endpoint of osteoporosis is fracture. The risk of sustaining a fracture in an individual is determined by the combination of the fragility of their bones and their risk of sustaining trauma, most commonly in the form of a fall. Variation in bone mineral density (BMD), as measured by dual-energy X-ray absorptiometry (DXA), accounts for 60–90% of the variation in bone fragility and is the most commonly used method of assessing a patient's future risk of fracture. Prospective population studies have demonstrated that for each standard deviation reduction in BMD there is an approximate doubling of the risk of sustaining a fracture. However, BMD is only one of many risk factors for fracture (**Table 3.1**). This chapter discusses the spectrum of risk factors for fracture and their use in more detail.

Age and gender

Age and gender are two of the strongest predictors of an individual's risk for fracture. Appendicular fractures exhibit a bimodal distribution, with an initial peak at 10–20 years that is generally attributed to traumatic fractures. The second peak in people aged >50 years corresponds to lower trauma fractures that are generally assumed to be osteoporotic in nature (**Figure 3.1**) [1]. The second peak demonstrates a much higher rate of fracture in females compared with males at any given age: 80% of hip fractures occur in women, 90% occur in patients aged >50 years, and 52% in those aged >80 years.

Although age and sex are not modifiable, they are important variables in determining an individual's risk of fracture in the short- to medium-term. A 50-year-old man has a 0.84% chance of sustaining a hip fracture in the next 10 years of life compared with an 18% risk in an 80-year-old woman (**Table 3.2**) [2]. A patient's age and sex should therefore form an integral part of assessing the fracture risk, and should be used in combination with other risk factors in deciding on the level of therapeutic intervention required in an individual.

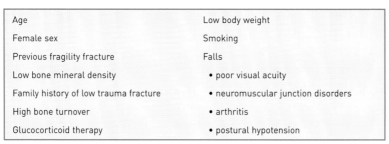

Age	Low body weight
Female sex	Smoking
Previous fragility fracture	Falls
Low bone mineral density	• poor visual acuity
Family history of low trauma fracture	• neuromuscular junction disorders
High bone turnover	• arthritis
Glucocorticoid therapy	• postural hypotension

Table 3.1 Risk factors for osteoporotic fracture.

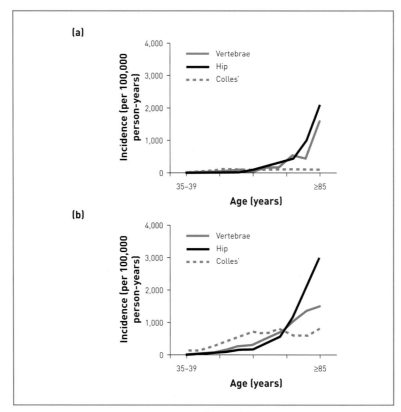

Figure 3.1 Incidence of fractures by age and sex: **(a)** men, **(b)** women. Reproduced from *J Bone Miner Res* 1992;7:221–7 with permission of the American Society for Bone and Mineral Research [1].

	Age (years)			
	50	60	70	80
Relative risk for hip fracture				
Men				
1	0.84	1.25	3.68	9.53
2	1.68	2.50	7.21	17.89
3	2.51	3.73	10.59	25.26
4	3.33	4.94	13.83	31.75
Women				
1	0.57	2.40	7.87	18.0
2	1.14	4.75	15.1	32.0
3	1.71	7.04	21.7	42.9
4	2.27	9.27	27.7	51.5
Hip, clinical spine, humeral, or Colles' fracture				
Men				
1	3.3	4.7	7.0	12.5
2	6.5	9.1	13.5	23.1
3	9.6	13.3	19.4	13.9
4	12.6	17.3	24.9	39.3
Women				
1	5.8	9.5	16.1	21.5
2	11.3	18.2	29.4	37.4
3	16.5	26.0	40.0	49.2
4	21.4	33.1	49.5	58.1

Table 3.2 Ten-year probability of fracture in men and women according to age and gender. Reproduced with permission from Elsevier [2].

Prior fracture

It has long been apparent that patients who have already sustained one fracture appear to be at a greater risk of subsequent fractures. This has now been confirmed in a number of epidemiologic studies, including several large cohort studies. These have been summarized in a statistical synthesis, which confirmed an approximate doubling of fractures at any site for a patient who had already sustained a previous fracture [3]. More interesting information can be gained by looking at site-specific fractures, which show that a fracture at any specific site has the greatest predictive value for fractures at that same site, although still predicting fractures at any of the classic osteoporotic sites (**Table 3.3**).

Prior fracture	Subsequent fracture (relative risk)			
	Wrist	**Hip**	**Vertebral**	**Any**
Wrist	3.3	1.9	1.7	2.0
Vertebral	1.4	2.3	4.4	1.9
Hip	–	2.3	2.5	2.4
Pooled	1.9	2.0	2.0	2.0

Table 3.3 The risk of fracture in postmenopausal women with a prior fracture.

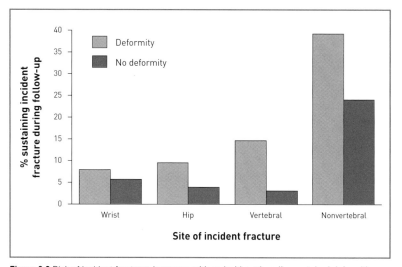

Figure 3.2 Risk of incident fractures in women with and without baseline vertebral deformities.

For example, a prior vertebral fracture increases the risk of a subsequent vertebral fracture by 4.4-fold. **Table 3.3** shows the data for postmenopausal women. Similar values are obtained for men and premenopausal women.

More information is available for vertebral fractures, where it is clear that with increasing severity of a vertebral fracture, as defined by loss of vertebral height or increasing number of vertebral fractures, the risk of sustaining a future fracture is dramatically increased (**Figure 3.2**) [4]. One obvious explanation for this increased risk would be that these patients have low BMD and hence have a greater subsequent fracture risk. However, a number of studies have examined this by adjusting for BMD at baseline. They found that the increased risk of fracture, and, interestingly, the increasing risk with the increasing number of vertebral fractures, remains both clinically and statistically significant after adjustment for BMD. It is therefore likely that the increased risk is due to other

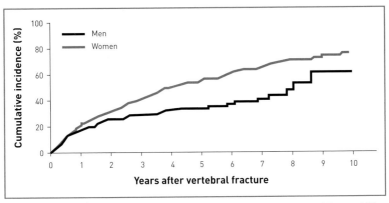

Figure 3.3 Risk of subsequent fracture after initial vertebral fracture. Data from Melton et al [5].

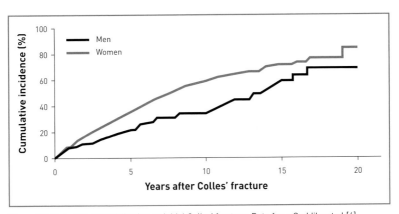

Figure 3.4 Risk of fracture following an initial Colles' fracture. Data from Cuddihy et al [6].

nondensitometric factors such as bone geometry and microarchitecture, and possibly the risk of falling.

Of most clinical importance is the immediacy of this increased risk. Cohort studies following patients who have sustained vertebral fractures have demonstrated that 20% will sustain a subsequent fracture within 1 year of their initial vertebral fracture, rising to 60% at 5 years for women and just under 40% at 5 years for men (**Figure 3.3**) [5]. **Figure 3.4** demonstrates similar data, showing an extremely high risk of fracture in the first few years following an initial Colles' fracture [6]. These studies confirm the importance of identifying and treating patients with osteoporotic fractures as a matter of priority.

BMD measurement	Future fracture (relative risk)			
	Forearm	Hip	Vertebral	Any
Distal radius BMD	1.7	1.8	1.7	1.4
Femoral neck BMD	1.4	2.6	1.8	1.6
Lumbar spine BMD	1.5	1.6	2.3	1.5

Table 3.4 Relative risks of fracture in women per standard deviation decrease in bone mineral density (BMD).

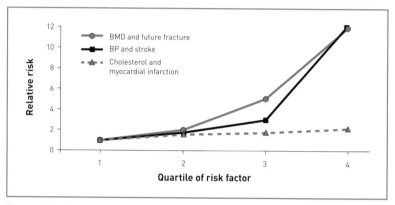

Figure 3.5 Risk factors for selected chronic diseases.

Bone mineral density

An estimate of BMD obtained from DXA scans has been shown to be strongly predictive of future fractures. For each standard deviation below baseline measurements in BMD, there is an approximate doubling of the risk of future fracture [7]. Although BMD taken at any site is predictive of any osteoporotic fracture, BMD measured at the site of interest is usually the best predictive factor (**Table 3.4**). The association between BMD and future fracture is of equivalent strength to the association between hypertension and stroke, and significantly greater than that of the association between hypercholesterolemia and myocardial infarction (**Figure 3.5**).

BMD is therefore a good predictor of future fracture, but, as with the use of hypertension in predicting stroke, it should be used as a strong predictor of fracture in combination with other risk factors rather than as the sole diagnostic criterion for osteoporosis. BMD can be used to estimate a patient's individual lifetime risk of fracture: depending on BMD, a 50-year-old white woman's lifetime risk of fracture can be estimated at between 5 and 50% (**Figure 3.6**) [8]. Calculations of 5- and 10-year absolute risk of fracture by age, sex, and BMD would lead to greater clinical utility and should be available in the near future.

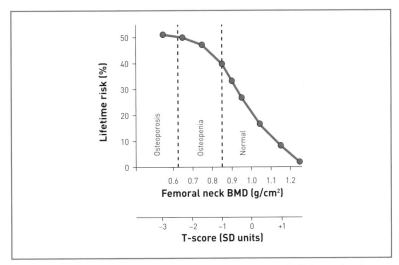

Figure 3.6 Lifetime risk of hip fracture in 50-year-old Swedish women. BMD: bone mineral density; SD: standard deviation. Reproduced with permission from Elsevier [2].

Female sex	Family history of hip fracture[a]
Premature menopause	Poor visual acuity[a]
Age[a]	Low body weight[a]
Primary or secondary amenorrhea	Neuromuscular disorders[a]
Primary and secondary hypogonadism in men	Cigarette smoking[a]
Asian or white ethnic origin	Excessive alcohol consumption
Previous fragility fracture[a]	Long-term immobilization
Low bone mineral density	Low dietary calcium intake
Glucocorticoid therapy[a]	Vitamin D deficiency
High bone turnover[a]	

Table 3.5 Indications for bone densitometry. [a]Characteristics that capture aspects of fracture risk over and above that provided by bone mineral density.

Risk factors for low BMD

Although BMD is strongly associated with future fracture risk, it is not advocated as a population screening tool. This is due to its relatively low sensitivity to predict fracture: although patients with a T-score of below –2.5 have a high risk of fracture, a large number of fractures occur in those with a BMD above this level. A case-finding strategy is therefore recommended (see **Chapter 4**), whereby patients deemed to be at high risk of osteoporosis based on clinical risk factors are advised to undergo assessment of BMD (**Table 3.5**, **Figure 3.7**).

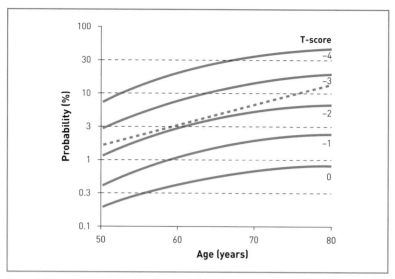

Figure 3.7 Ten-year probability of hip fracture in Swedish men and women, according to T-scores assessed at the femoral neck by dual-energy X-ray absorptiometry. Probability scale is logarithmic. The brown dotted line represents the probability at which interventions are cost-effective. Reproduced with permission from Elsevier [2].

Genetics

A genetic component to osteoporosis has been suspected for many years, but it was not until the development of reproducible techniques for measuring BMD that this was confirmed or quantified. The majority of work has come from twin and family studies. A large number of studies have concentrated on peak bone mass in females and have shown remarkably consistent results. Heritability estimates, defined as a proportion of the population variance attributable to genetic factors, range from 0.42 to 0.98 and are consistent in studies from several different continents. In studies where BMD has been measured at multiple sites, there seems to be a consistent trend for greater heritability in the lumbar spine, with lower estimates at appendicular sites such as the distal and mid-shaft of the radius and femoral neck (**Figure 3.8**).

Twin studies examining postmenopausal bone density, which reflects a combination of peak bone mass and postmenopausal bone loss, still demonstrate a significant genetic component, although somewhat lower than that of the peak bone mass, with heritability estimates ranging from 0.46 to 0.84 [9]. This would imply that postmenopausal bone loss has a lower genetic component than peak bone mass.

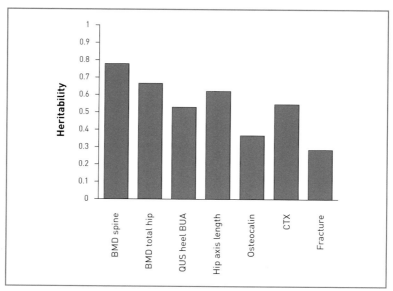

Figure 3.8 Heritability of bone density, structure, and metabolism. BMD: bone mineral density; BUA: broadband ultrasound attenuation; CTX: urinary type I C-telopeptide; QUS: quantitative ultrasound.

This has been addressed in two studies. A small study of 40 Australian twin pairs that examined the heritability of change in bone mass over 3 years found a genetic component to lumbar spine change, but not femoral neck [10]. Unfortunately, there were not enough postmenopausal twins to assess postmenopausal bone loss directly. A second study of male twin pairs followed up for 16 years found no significant genetic component of bone loss at the mid-radius [11].

Genetic factors of other aspects of bone metabolism and geometry

Although BMD is the main predictor of bone strength and fracture risk, two other measurements deserve mention at this point: quantitative ultrasound of the calcaneous and hip axis length.

Broadband ultrasound attenuation (BUA), velocity of sound (VOS), and stiffness can be assessed from heel quantitative ultrasound measurements, and have been shown to be associated with fractures with a relative risk of approximately 2 for each standard deviation decrease in BUA and VOS. This association is independent of their known correlation with BMD, suggesting that they may measure structural properties of bone not detected by DXA. A large study of postmenopausal white twins has demonstrated a moderate genetic component to both of these parameters, with heritability estimates of 0.53 for BUA and 0.58 for VOS [9]. This component was not significantly reduced when

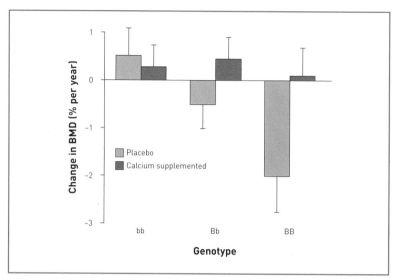

Figure 3.9 Adjusted rates of bone mineral density (BMD) change by vertebral disc ratio at the femoral neck in 229 healthy postmenopausal women participating in a placebo-controlled trial of calcium supplementation with 500 mg of elemental calcium. Reproduced from *J Bone Miner Res* 1995;10:978–84 with permission of the American Society for Bone and Mineral Research [13].

adjusted for BMD, further supporting a genetic component to other aspects of bone strength independent of BMD.

The same study examined the heritability of hip axis length (the distance from the greater trochanter, through the femoral neck, to the inner rim of the acetabulum), which is an independent predictor of hip fracture with an increased risk of 1.7 for every standard deviation increase in length. This again had a moderate genetic component, with a heritability estimate of 0.62 independent of height, suggesting a local effect on hip geometry rather than on simple body size alone [9].

Bone metabolism, as assessed by biochemical markers of bone resorption and formation, has also been assessed for a genetic component [12]. Bone resorption, (assessed by urinary amino-terminal collagen type-I telopeptide) and bone formation (assessed by serum osteocalcin) have moderate genetic components, with heritability estimates of 0.55 and 0.37, respectively.

Which genes are responsible?

Genetic modeling has suggested that most of these traits are polygenic, with a number of different genes involved. Numerous genes have been examined and several found to be associated with BMD and other markers of bone metabolism; however, few have been found to explain more than a small proportion of their overall variance. Those with positive associations to date include genes for the vitamin D receptor, estrogen receptor, insulin-like growth factor (IGF)-1, growth hormone, and type I collagen.

The reasons for this failure to find genes displaying a major genetic component may in part be due to the current polymorphisms being identified, which are often not functional and are probably in linkage disequilibrium with more important genes. In addition, the genome is unlikely to work in isolation from the environment. Several important environmental genetic interactions have already been demonstrated, and many more have yet to be discovered (**Figure 3.9**) [13]. Further refinement of the genome screen and the search for more important environmental genetic interactions will eventually shed more light on this important area of research.

Genetics of fracture

Support for a genetic component to osteoporotic fracture comes from studies that have demonstrated that a family history of fracture increases an individual's risk of sustaining an osteoporotic fracture. A large cohort study of American women aged ≥65 years demonstrated that a maternal history of hip fracture was associated with a doubling of the risk of sustaining a hip fracture [14]. Furthermore, a large UK case-control study found that a history of a female relative with a previous Colles' fracture doubled the risk of osteoporotic fracture, and increased the risk of a Colles' fracture by 4-fold [15]. In both of these cases, the increased risk of fracture was independent of BMD, suggesting that factors other than bone mass are involved.

A large prospective study of male and female twins from Finland has directly examined the heritability of fracture [16]. The authors concluded that the genetic component of fracture was relatively small at <30%, and appeared to be smaller in women than in men. Although there is a genetic component to osteoporotic fractures, it is much smaller than that of BMD. As fracture is the end result of a number of factors (including BMD, turnover, body size and shape, muscle function, and the risk of falling), which are all controlled by different genetic pathways, it is difficult to disentangle the genetics of fracture. Furthermore, there are a host of important environmental factors operating, which will almost certainly interact with the genome. The challenge for the future is to discover how environmental factors and the genome interact to fully determine the risk of fracture.

Biochemical markers of bone turnover

An increasing range of biochemical markers of both bone formation and bone resorption is now available for research, and increasingly for clinical applications (see **Chapter 6**). It is well accepted that these markers increase at the time of the menopause, associated with increased rates of bone loss. Several studies have looked at the ability of biochemical markers to predict rates of bone loss, with disparate results. Those that have followed patients in the long term do tend to suggest that high rates of bone resorption are associated with increased rates of bone loss.

A more important question is whether they predict fracture risk. Several large cohort studies have now demonstrated that patients with high rates of bone turnover, as assessed by free deoxypyridinoline and urinary type 1 C-telopeptide (CTX), are associated with an increased risk of hip fracture [17]. The risks provided by these assessments appear to be less marked than those for BMD. However, they do appear to be independent of BMD and therefore may add extra information. Garnero et al. found that a combination of high CTX and low BMD gave an odds ratio of 4.8 for hip fracture in elderly women [18].

Under-carboxylated osteocalcin has also been shown to predict hip fracture risk, with raised values being associated with an odds ratio of 1.9 [19]. This study, again, showed that combining the lowest quartile of BMD with the highest quartile of under-carboxylated osteocalcin increased the odds ratio of fracture to 5.5.

These results suggest that combining markers of bone turnover with BMD estimation may improve our ability to predict fracture, although further work is still required to define the most suitable marker to be used and its relevant threshold.

Corticosteroids

It has long been accepted that both endogenous hypercortisolism and exogenous corticosteroid administration are associated with an increased risk of osteoporosis. Corticosteroid therapy is an important risk factor to consider when assessing fracture risk, as there are an estimated 350,000 patients in the UK taking oral corticosteroids, and up to 25% of cases of osteoporosis are at least partially attributable to corticosteroid therapy [20].

Corticosteroid therapy-induced bone loss is greatest during the first year of therapy, and data have demonstrated that there is also a rapid increase in fracture risk, which is present within the first few months of therapy [21] (see **Chapter 9** for a more comprehensive discussion of corticosteroids and osteoporosis). Prednisolone doses of <7.5 mg/day were traditionally thought to be 'safe' for bone health. However, more recent data have demonstrated that vertebral fracture risk is increased at doses as low as 2.5 mg/day, with increases in hip fracture risk at doses of 2.5–5 mg/day. The risk of fracture increases in a dose-dependent fashion at all sites with increasing doses of corticosteroids (**Figure 3.10**) [21]. The prevalence and dosage of corticosteroid therapy is greatest in the elderly, who are already at a high risk of osteoporotic fracture, making them a priority for management.

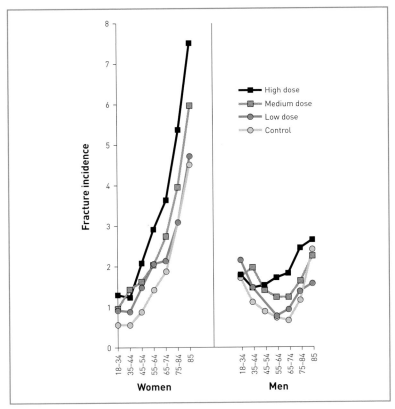

Figure 3.10 Incidence of nonvertebral fractures stratified by daily corticosteroid dose, age, and gender. Reproduced from *J Bone Miner Res* 2000:15:993–1000 with permission of the American Society for Bone and Mineral Research [21].

Patients taking inhaled corticosteroids are also at an increased risk of fracture, although their risk is not significantly different from that of patients with respiratory disease who are not using inhaled corticosteroids. It is therefore uncertain whether inhaled corticosteroids do increase the risk of fracture or whether the increased risk is due to the disease itself. Patients on high-dose inhaled corticosteroids (0.8 mg/day of beclomethasone dipropionate) should be fully assessed for osteoporosis, as there may be an increased risk of fracture.

Estimation of fracture risk

The estimation of BMD forms an integral part of the assessment of fracture risk. It has been suggested that, for any given value of BMD, patients on oral corticosteroids are more likely to sustain a fracture [22,23]. Also, the increased fracture risk is independent of BMD due to the effects of corticosteroids on nondensitometric risk factors for fracture, such as bone quality and fall risk.

Source	Amount	Vitamin D (µg)
Milk, whole	190 mL (1/3 pt)	0.06
Milk, semi-skimmed	190 mL (1/3 pt)	0.02
Milk, skimmed	190 mL (1/3 pt)	Trace
Cheddar cheese	100 g (3½ oz)	0.26
Eggs	100 g (3½ oz)	1.75
Butter	100 g (3½ oz)	0.76
Margarine (fortified)	100 g (3½ oz)	7.15
Liver (raw)	100 g (3½ oz)	4.50
Tuna (canned)	100 g (3½ oz)	5.80
Pacific salmon (raw)	100 g (3½ oz)	12.50

Table 3.6 Dietary sources of vitamin D. Recommended daily amount = 400 IU/day (10 µg).

It has therefore been suggested that for patients on oral corticosteroids, a T-score of −1.5 or −1.0 should be used as a diagnostic threshold.

It is important not to forget the underlying disease process in patients on oral corticosteroids. In many of the inflammatory diseases in which corticosteroids are used (eg, rheumatoid arthritis and inflammatory bowel disease), the inflammatory process itself may lead to bone loss and an increased risk of fracture [24]. Wherever possible, the disease should be controlled using steroid-sparing therapies or by alternative routes for steroid administration, such as intra-articular therapies and enemas. Furthermore, diseases such as rheumatoid arthritis and myasthenia gravis are associated with an increased risk of falling, and a full assessment of fall risk should be performed.

Corticosteroid therapy is associated with a substantial and rapid increase in the risk of fracture, and patients commencing, or currently receiving, corticosteroid therapy should be regarded as high risk and assessed as a matter of priority.

Diet and other lifestyle factors

Calcium
Calcium is one of the most important constituents of bone, with 97% of total body calcium held in the skeleton. The ability of the intestine to absorb dietary calcium decreases with age, with the most pronounced decrements after the menopause and after the age of 70 years. In a large cohort study of women >65 years, low intestinal absorption of calcium was shown to predict hip fracture [25]. Furthermore, dietary calcium intake is often low in the elderly population.

Although the association of calcium intake and osteoporosis has been inconsistent in epidemiologic studies, a meta-analysis of retrospective studies

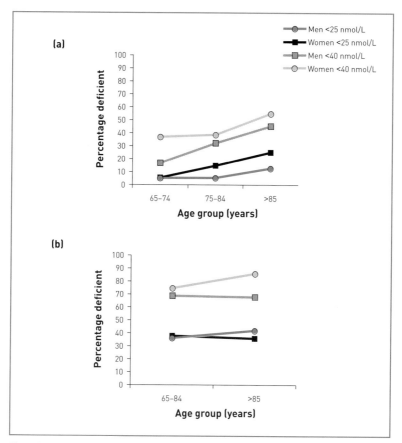

Figure 3.11 Vitamin D deficiency in **(a)** free-living and **(b)** institutionalized men and women.

demonstrated a positive association between calcium intake and BMD [26]. Clinical trials have demonstrated that calcium supplementation leads to an increased BMD and reduced fracture risk, particularly in those with low calcium intake [27].

Vitamin D

Vitamin D is integrally involved in bone metabolism through stimulation of calcium absorption from the intestine and resorption from the kidneys. It also has direct effects on osteoclasts, as well as indirect effects through secondary hyperparathyroidism. In young adults, most circulating vitamin D is produced in the skin following exposure to sunlight. However, with aging, the ability of the skin to produce vitamin D is reduced, as is the amount of exposure to sunlight, such that we become dependent on dietary sources of vitamin D to maintain adequate vitamin D stores (**Table 3.6**).

Previous fall	Parkinson's disease
Poor visual acuity	Myasthenia gravis
Reduced depth perception	Postural hypotension
Reduced muscle strength (inability to rise from a chair)	Drug therapy
	Long-acting benzodiazepines
Balance or gait deficit	Antihypertensive agents
Diseases leading to impaired neuromuscular function	Polypharmacy (greater than four drugs)
Arthritis	Environmental hazards around the home
Stroke	

Table 3.7 Risk factors for nonsyncopal falls.

Vitamin D deficiency is common in the elderly, particularly those who are in institutions (**Figure 3.11**). Approximately one-third of free-living individuals aged >75 years and two-thirds of institutionalized individuals aged ≥65 years are biochemically deficient in vitamin D [28]. These individuals will most probably have secondary hyperparathyroidism, with its associated increased rates of bone loss. Supplementation of elderly patients with vitamin D, often with calcium, can reverse secondary hyperparathyroidism, increase BMD, and reduce the risk of fracture [29,30]. The relative importance of calcium and vitamin D supplementation in these studies is currently uncertain; however, trials set to answer this question should report within the next 2 years. In the meantime, it seems sensible to assess and correct dietary calcium and vitamin D deficiency in individuals at risk of fracture.

Other dietary factors

Numerous dietary constituents have been associated with low BMD, although results are often inconsistent due to limitations of assessment of dietary intakes. The most important limitation in the analysis of micronutrient intake is that several micronutrients are often contained in certain food types, making it impossible to differentiate between them in any analysis. It may therefore be more sensible to assess dietary patterns of eating, rather than individual micronutrients, when looking for associations with osteoporosis.

Dietary factors that tend to be associated with reduced BMD include: high intake of caffeine-containing drinks; high protein intake; low vitamin K intake; and alcoholism. As these factors often affect fracture risk through BMD, and their effects are small, it is unlikely that they will add significantly to the assessment of fracture risk if an estimate of BMD has already been obtained.

Low body weight

Low body weight, and in particular low body mass index, is strongly associated with a reduction in BMD and an increased risk of fracture. Patients with anorexia nervosa have reduced BMD and an increased risk of fracture. The association between weight and BMD remains strong, even within the normal ranges of body weight, and is consistent across the different sites of BMD measured [31]. There are several potential mechanisms to explain the increased fracture risk in individuals with low body weight, including:

- decreased mechanical loading of bone
- hypogonadism
- reduced production of estrone in adipocytes
- low insulin and IGF-I concentrations
- (for hip fracture) less impact-absorbing fatty padding over the greater trochanter

Smoking

Smoking tobacco reduces BMD by several mechanisms: altered metabolism of sex hormones and hormone replacement therapy, an earlier menopause, reduced intestinal calcium absorption, and reduced body weight. There is an increased risk of fracture; however, this is relatively small and adds little once an estimate of BMD has been obtained.

Falls

Although 90% of hip fractures are the result of a fall from standing height or less, only 1% of falls result in a hip fracture. Falls that result in a hip fracture tend to occur on a hard surface, with the patient falling straight down or sideways, landing directly on the hip.

Of these falls:

- 50% are the result of slipping or tripping
- 20% are due to syncope
- 13–20% are due to loss of balance
- the rest are due to miscellaneous factors [32]

Falls occur with increasing frequency with aging, and much is now known about the risk factors for recurrent falling (**Table 3.7**). Many of these risk factors are correctable (visual impairment, polypharmacy, muscle weakness), and early trials suggest that targeted single or multiple interventions can reduce the risk of falls [33,34].

Conclusion

When faced with a patient in the clinic, it is important to try to assess their risk of fracture in order to decide on the appropriate level of therapeutic intervention. This assessment should be based on a combination of risk factors and not just the patient's BMD estimation. Ideally, the risk of sustaining an osteoporotic fracture in the next 5–10 years should be estimated. Although, it is not possible to do this accurately with currently available data, a reasonable estimate can be made.

Using the data from Sweden and by knowing the patient's age and gender, we can estimate the baseline risk of hip or any other fracture at the classic osteoporotic site (**Table 3.2**). If there is a clinical indication to estimate BMD (**Table 3.5**), ideally, this should be performed at the lumbar spine and hip. For each standard deviation that the BMD lies below the young adult mean (T-score), the risk of fracture is approximately doubled; and, therefore, the risk for that patient can be computed from their BMD, age, and gender. Other risk factors can then be built into this model; however, if a risk factor exerts its effect exclusively through reduced BMD, it will add no further information to the model. Risk factors that exert part of their effect through BMD will add less to the model than anticipated, and the relative risk should be reduced accordingly. The level of risk that justifies treatment will depend on the health economics of the relevant healthcare system. If the BMD value is not available, an estimate of risk can be produced from clinical risk factors alone. Caution should be used with this approach, however, if it is used to make decisions regarding therapeutic interventions. An elderly person with poor vision, poor gait, muscle weakness, and postural hypotension may produce an absolute risk of hip fracture to justify administering bisphosphonates on health economic grounds, but would obviously be much better served by a referral to a specialist falls service.

There are some exceptions to this approach, including corticosteroid-induced osteoporosis, where specific guidelines exist for management of these patients. Patients with an existing osteoporotic fracture are at a particularly high risk of future fracture and should be treated in all but rare circumstances.

References

1. Cooper C, Atkinson EJ, O'Fallon WM, et al. Incidence of clinically diagnosed vertebral fractures: a population-based study in Rochester, Minnesota, 1985–89. *J Bone Miner Res* 1992;7:221–7.

2. Kanis JA. Diagnosis of osteoporosis and assessment of fracture risk. *Lancet* 2002;359:1929–36.

3. Klotzbuecher CM, Ross PD, Landsman PB, et al. Patients with prior fractures have an increased risk of future fractures: a summary of the literature and statistical synthesis. *J Bone Miner Res* 2000;15:721–39.

4. Black DM, Arden NK, Palermo L, et al. Prevalent vertebral deformities predict hip fractures and new vertebral deformities but not wrist fractures. Study of osteoporotic fractures research group. *J Bone Miner Res* 1999;14:821–8.

5. Melton LJ III, Atkinson EJ, Cooper C, et al. Vertebral fractures predict subsequent fractures. *Osteoporos Int* 1999;10:214–21.

6. Cuddihy MT, Gabriel, SE, Crowson CS, et al. Forearm fractures as predictors of subsequent osteoporotic fractures. *Osteoporos Int* 1999;9:469–75.

7. Marshall, D, Johnell O, Wedel H. Meta-analysis of how well measures of bone mineral density predict occurrence of osteoporotic fractures. *BMJ* 1996;312:1254–9.

8. Kanis JA, Glüer C-C. An update on the diagnosis and assessment of osteoporosis with densitometry. Committee of Scientific Advisors, International Osteoporosis Foundation. *Osteoporos Int* 2000;11:192–202.

9. Arden NK, Baker J, Hogg C, et al. The heritability of bone mineral density, ultrasound of the calcaneus and hip axis length: a study of postmenopausal twins. *J Bone Miner Res* 1996;11:530–4.

10. Kelly PJ, Nguyen T, Hopper J, et al. Changes in axial bone density with age: a twin study. *J Bone Miner Res* 1993;8:11–17.

11. Slemenda CW, Christian JC, Reed T, et al. Long-term bone loss in men: effects of genetic and environmental factors. *Ann Intern Med* 1992;117:286–91.

12. Garnero P, Arden NK, Griffiths G, et al. Genetic influence on bone turnover in postmenopausal twins. *J Clin Endocrinol Metab* 1996;81:140–6.

13. Krall EA, Parry P, Lichter JB, et al. Vitamin D receptor alleles and rates of bone loss: influences of years since menopause and calcium intake. *J Bone Miner Res* 1995;10:978–84.

14. Cummings SR, Nevitt MC, Browner WS et al. Risk factors for hip fracture in white women. Study of osteoporotic fractures research group. *N Engl J Med* 1995;332:767–73.

15. Keen RW, Hart DJ, Arden NK, et al. Family history of appendicular fracture and risk of osteoporosis: a population-based study. *Osteoporos Int* 1999;10:161–6.

16. Kannus P, Palvanen M, Kaprio J, et al. Genetic factors and osteoporotic fractures in elderly people: prospective 25 year follow up of a nationwide cohort of elderly Finnish twins. *BMJ* 1999;319:1334–7.

17. Garnero P, Hausherr E, Chapuy MC, et al. Markers of bone resorption predict hip fracture in elderly women: the EPIDOS Prospective Study. *J Bone Miner Res* 1996;11:1531–8.

18. Garnero P, Sornay-Rendu E, Chapuy MC, et al. Increased bone turnover in late postmenopausal women is a major determinant of osteoporosis. *J Bone Miner Res* 1996;11:337–49.

19. Vergnaud P, Garnero P, Meunier PJ, et al. Undercarboxylated osteocalcin measured with a specific immunoassay predicts hip fracture in elderly women: the EPIDOS Study. *J Clin Endocrinol Metab* 1997;82:719–24.

20. Compston JE, Barlow D, Brown P, et al. Glucocorticoid - induced osteoporosis – guidelines for prevention and treatment. London: Royal College of Physicians, 2002.

21. Van Staa TP, Leufkens HG, Abenhaim L, et al. Use of oral corticosteroids and risk of fractures. *J Bone Miner Res* 2000;15:993–1000.

22. Luengo M, Picado C, Del Rio L, et al. Vertebral fractures in steroid dependent asthma and involutional osteoporosis: a comparative study. *Thorax* 1991;46:803–6.

23. Peel NF, Moore DJ, Barrington NA, et al. Risk of vertebral fracture and relationship to bone mineral density in steroid treated rheumatoid arthritis. *Ann Rheum Dis* 1995;54:801–6.

24. Van Staa TP, Cooper C, Brusse LS, et al. Inflammatory bowel disease and the risk of fracture. *Gastroenterology* 2003;125:1591–7.

25. Ensrud KE, Duong T, Cauley JA, et al. Low fractional calcium absorption increases the risk for hip fracture in women with low calcium intake. Study of Osteoporotic Fractures Research Group. *Ann Intern Med* 2000;132:345–53.

26. Cumming RG. Calcium intake and bone mass: a quantitative review of the evidence. *Calcif Tissue Int* 1990;47:194–201.

27. Dawson-Hughes B, Dallal GE, Krall EA, et al. Controlled trial of the effect of calcium supplementation on bone density in postmenopausal women. *N Engl J Med* 1990;323:878–83.

28. Royal College of Physicians, Bone and Tooth Society of Great Britain, National Osteoporosis Society. *Glucocorticoid-induced osteoporosis. Guidelines for prevention and treatment.* London: Royal College of Physicians of London, 2002.

29. Finch S, Doyle W, Lowe C, et al. National Diet and Nutritional Survey: People aged 65 years and over. Volume 1. *Report of the Diet and Nutrition Survey.* London: HMSO, 1998.

30. Dawson-Hughes B. Bone loss accompanying medical therapies. *N Engl J Med* 2001;345:989–91.

31. Chapuy MC, Arlot ME, Duboeuf F, et al. Vitamin D3 and calcium to prevent hip fractures in the elderly women. *N Engl J Med* 1992;327:1637–42.

32. Dawson-Hughes B, Shipp C, Sadowski L, et al. Bone density of the radius, spine, and hip in relation to percent of ideal body weight in postmenopausal women. *Calcif Tissue Int* 1987;40:310–4.

33. Nevitt MC, Cummings SR. Type of fall and risk of hip and wrist fractures: the Study of Osteoporotic Fractures. The Study of Osteoporotic Fractures Research Group. *J Am Geriatr Soc* 1993;41:1226–34.

34. Tinetti ME. Clinical practice. Preventing falls in elderly persons. *N Engl J Med* 2003;348:42–9.

35. American Geriatrics Society, British Geriatrics Society, and American Academy of Orthopaedic Surgeons. Guideline for the prevention of falls in older persons. *J Am Geriatr Soc* 2001;49:664–72.

4

Strategies for the Prevention and Management of Osteoporosis

Pam Brown

Introduction

Osteoporosis is defined as a "progressive systemic skeletal disease characterized by low bone mass and microarchitectural deterioration of bone tissue, with a consequent increase in bone fragility and susceptibility to fracture" [1].

Osteoporosis is a silent disease until the first fracture occurs – the clinical significance of osteoporosis lies in the fractures that it causes. A total of 10% of women over the age of 70 years will suffer a hip fracture in any 5-year period, 10–20% will die as a result, and 50% of the survivors will require long-term care [2]. The goal of prevention is therefore to prevent first and subsequent fractures, particularly hip fractures. As with any chronic disease, several different strategies can be used to tackle the disease, and these are outlined in **Table 4.1**. The aim is to reduce fractures while making the most cost-effective use of resources.

Osteoporosis can be tackled predominantly in primary care, although investigation and treatment can be initiated in secondary care with primary care follow-up. Patient education and involvement of a multidisciplinary team are vital for both approaches.

Each strategy is discussed here, while the reader is referred to other chapters for further details of specific diagnostic tools, high-risk groups, and treatments.

Population strategies

Two types of population-based strategy exist. In the first, attempts are made to decrease fracture risk by improving the bone mineral density (BMD) of the whole population. In the second strategy, a subpopulation is screened to identify those with osteoporosis, or those who are at risk of developing it, and these high-risk individuals are offered treatment.

Strategies
Population strategies:
Improve bone mineral density across the whole population
Population screening
Selective case-finding (high-risk) strategies:
Opportunistic identification of high-risk individuals
'Search and rescue' strategies for high-risk groups
Organizational issues
Primary prevention versus secondary prevention
Primary care versus shared secondary/primary care

Table 4.1 Approaches to the prevention and treatment of osteoporosis.

Improving BMD across the whole population

A 10% increase in average female BMD would halve osteoporotic fractures [3]. Such a strategy would need to target all ages, encouraging lifelong change (a 'cradle to the grave' approach), and would be time-consuming to implement; compliance is likely to be poor. However, lifestyle advice to improve bone health is similar to that used to reduce coronary heart disease, stroke, diabetes, and cancer (**Table 4.2**). Healthcare providers deliver this advice already; adding bone benefits to the messages may make some impact. There is little evidence from intervention studies that improving lifestyle reduces fractures, so it is clear this should not be the only strategy used to reduce fracture risk.

Exercise

Exercise can increase BMD in adults by 1–5% [4], with a significant impact on fracture risk; the benefit reverses once exercise stops [5]. Epidemiologic studies suggest that active lifestyles may reduce hip fracture risk, but that the type of exercise is important [5]. Although, conventionally, weight-bearing exercise is recommended, low-impact exercise such as walking does not improve bone mass [5], while high-impact exercise such as jogging or jumping does. Slow lifting of heavy weights (70–85% personal maximum) can also increase BMD in both pre- and postmenopausal women [5,6], but this is not appropriate for those with previous vertebral fractures.

Exercise improves postural stability and reduces falls in the elderly [7]. Walking improves mobility and general health, but does not improve falls risk, and may increase fracture risk [8]. The Frailty and Injuries: Cooperative Studies of Intervention Techniques (FICSIT) meta-analysis showed a 10% reduction in falls in the intervention groups, with a 50% reduction with a Tai Chi program [9], and a significant fall reduction with individually tailored, supervised programs [10].

Well-balanced diet containing adequate protein and calories
Five portions of fruit and vegetables daily
Low sodium and high potassium intake
>800 mg calcium daily
Adequate vitamin D from diet and/or sunlight
<300 mg caffeine daily (three cups of brewed coffee, six cans of caffeinated beverages)
Weight-bearing and resistance exercise to improve bone mineral density
Exercise to improve postural stability, eg, Tai Chi
Smoking cessation
Falls prevention assessment, if appropriate

Table 4.2 Summary of lifestyle recommendations for optimizing bone mass and preventing fractures.

Diet

In common with many other diseases, adopting a healthy, balanced diet is important in the prevention of osteoporosis. Anorexia nervosa is associated with a reduced BMD and an increased risk of fracture. Certain components of the diet merit particular attention. Vitamin D is important throughout life for optimal calcium absorption and bone metabolism. A dietary survey has shown that adolescents and the elderly are most at risk of vitamin D insufficiency and deficiency. Eleven per cent of 11- to 14-year-olds, and 16% of boys and 10% of girls aged 15–18 years were found to have vitamin D-deficient diets [11]. Most of the elderly surveyed had low dietary intakes of vitamin D, and 10% of community-dwelling and 37% of institutionalized elderly had low blood levels of vitamin D [12]. It is also important to maintain an adequate calcium intake, particularly in the young, who often prefer carbonated drinks to milk.

The Framingham Osteoporosis Study and other population-based studies have linked high intakes of potassium, magnesium, and vitamin K from fruit and vegetables with improved BMD and reduced hip fracture rates in the elderly [13–15]. The Framingham Osteoporosis Study demonstrated the highest rates of bone loss in those with the lowest protein intakes [16]. Protein intake is particularly important in improving outcome after hip fracture [17]. Since calcium and sodium are transported across the kidney tubule together, reducing sodium intake decreases urinary calcium excretion, but effects on BMD are unknown [4].

Some studies link high caffeine intake with reduced BMD [18] and/or increased hip fracture risk [19], although Harris and Dawson-Hughes found vertebral bone loss only in those with high caffeine intakes and low calcium intakes (440–744 mg/day) [20].

Alcohol
A modest intake of alcohol (1–2 drinks per day) may have beneficial effects on BMD. In women, this may relate to effects on adrenal androgens or estrogen concentrations. One study showed decreased fracture risk in drinkers versus nondrinkers [21], while an intake of >14 units of alcohol per week was associated with increased fracture risk [22].

Smoking
Smoking has little effect on premenopausal BMD; however, a meta-analysis demonstrated an increased risk of hip fracture in postmenopausal smokers, with a 19% cumulative hip fracture risk up to the age of 85 years in smokers compared with 12% in nonsmokers [23]. The risk decreases 5 years after smoking cessation in men, but not in women. Smoking may decrease the bone effects of hormone replacement therapy (HRT) by increasing the catabolism of estrogen and interfering with estrogen receptors.

Peak bone mass
Maximizing peak bone mass (PBM) should be a major focus of any population-based strategy. In growing children, calcium supplementation is associated with a 1–5% increase in bone mineral status, with maximum effects in the prepubertal period and early months of supplementation [24]. Supplementing with milk or dairy products may be better than with calcium alone, since milk-based protein may be independently beneficial to bone [25]. There appear to be threshold levels for calcium (eg, 1,400 mg/day in 2- to 8-year-olds), above which further intake does not increase PBM attained, but these levels are higher than recommended daily allowances and current average intakes.

Modest exercise during growth probably increases PBM, while excessive exercise, resulting in amenorrhea (female athlete triad), may be detrimental to PBM accumulation.

Population screening
A population screening approach using cheap and easily accessible investigations is successfully employed for coronary heart disease, hypertension, and diabetes. However, osteoporosis requires a dual-energy X-ray absorptiometry (DXA) scan for diagnosis, and this test is expensive, has low sensitivity, and is poor at predicting which patients will go on to fracture. Also, treatments for osteoporosis are not readily acceptable to many women. Screening populations of menopausal women with DXA and encouraging those identified as being at high risk to take HRT was undertaken in some centers in the UK, but was not cost effective. Population screening is therefore not currently recommended by the Royal College of Physicians in the UK [26], but DXA screening is being implemented in the USA.

A selective case-finding strategy is therefore recommended as the best method of identifying those at greatest risk, who require treatment to prevent fractures.

The remainder of this chapter addresses the practicalities of selective case finding in primary and secondary care, using opportunistic or 'search and rescue' approaches.

Selective case-finding strategies

Selective case-finding strategies rely on the use of risk factors and/or BMD to identify those at highest risk of future fracture. This identification process can take place opportunistically, or by undertaking specific searches for those with risk factors ('search and rescue' strategy). Some of these patients will be at very high risk of osteoporosis and can be treated, while others may require further investigation to establish their risk before treatment. All of those identified should be entered into a disease register.

Some of these people can be identified prior to their first fracture (primary prevention), while others will be identified at the time of their first fracture or later (secondary prevention).

Even though primary and secondary care teams diligently pursue a selective case-finding strategy, some patients will still develop fractures. For example, those without any of the conventional risk factors may not come to attention until they suffer their first fracture, and those who do not comply with therapy will continue to lose bone and suffer further fractures. Both groups can be identified when they fracture, and bone-preserving treatment can be initiated or restarted. This is discussed further in the next section.

Examples of selective case-finding opportunities are shown in **Table 4.3**. Groups at highest risk of future fracture, who should be targeted by the selective case-finding approach, are discussed in the next section.

Identifying groups at high risk of future fracture

Although osteoporosis can only be diagnosed using hip or spine DXA, several other factors can be used to predict future fracture risk. These include a history of previous fragility fracture, increasing age, the presence of other clinical risk factors or hip fracture risk factors, or low T-scores on ultrasound or peripheral DXA (pDXA). These risk factors for future fractures are listed in **Table 4.4** and discussed further in **Chapter 3**.

It is possible to combine risk factors to produce a 10-year prediction of fracture risk for individuals, in a similar way to the prediction of 10-year coronary heart disease risk, allowing drug treatment to be targeted to those at greatest risk [27]. One such score should be available in 2005. To achieve acceptable levels of predictive value when axial DXA is not available, it may be useful to combine, for example, clinical risk factors with quantitative ultrasound (QUS) or pDXA.

Risk factor	Method of identification	
	Primary care	Secondary care
Previous fragility fracture	Audit of women with previous hip fractures Hospital discharge letters Hospital clinic letters	Fracture initiatives (see below) Admissions
Oral steroid treatment	Audit of patients taking oral steroids Hospital discharge letters Hospital clinic letters	At treatment initiation
House-bound elderly	Computer search Opportunistically on house calls	At discharge to nursing and residential homes
Early menopause	Opportunistically in smear clinic	Discharge following hysterectomy/oophorectomy
Vertebral fracture	High index of suspicion in postmenopausal women with back pain	High awareness in radiologists reporting spinal X-rays

Table 4.3 Selective case finding in primary and secondary care. DXA: dual-energy X-ray absorptiometry.

Previous fragility fracture

Previous fracture since the age of 50 years greatly increases the risk of future fracture. Patients with a vertebral fracture have a 4.3 relative risk (RR) of further fracture if their BMD is normal, rising to an RR of 12.6 if they also have low BMD. This compares with a 2.5 RR with low BMD and no previous fracture. Of women with vertebral fracture, 20% refracture within 1 year without treatment; this group has a 3–5 times increased risk of future vertebral fracture, and twice the risk of any future fracture compared with women without prevalent vertebral fracture.

Oral glucocorticoid therapy

Oral glucocorticoid therapy at any dose, for 3 months or more, increases fracture risk. Patients >65 years or those with other risk factors (eg, previous fracture) should be started on bone-sparing therapy at the initiation of glucocorticoids [28]. Those <65 years need a DXA scan, and bone-sparing therapy should be initiated if the T score is –1.5 or below. Bone-sparing therapy can be started before DXA results if there is a delay, as bone is lost most rapidly during the first few months of glucocorticoid therapy.

Fallers

Although vertebral fractures may occur during normal activities such as bending or carrying, fragility wrist and hip fractures usually result from falls, making those who fall more likely to fracture. Those with a previous fall are more likely to sustain further falls. Identifying frequent fallers and enrolling them in a falls

Increasing age

Previous fragility fracture

Oral glucocorticoid use

High falls risk

Other clinical risk factors

- early menopause

- hyperthyroidism

Cummings' hip fracture risk factor score ≥5 (see text)

Low results on ultrasound scan or peripheral DXA

T-score <−2.5 on axial DXA

Table 4.4 Risk factors for future fracture. DXA: dual-energy X-ray absorptiometry.

prevention program may reduce their risk of subsequent falls. This is covered in more detail in **Chapter 3**.

Increasing age

Age is a strong risk factor for fracture risk. A 10-year increase in age increases hip fracture risk by 94% (for an average BMD decrease of 44% in elderly women) [29].

Axial DXA, pDXA, and QUS

Hip and spine DXA measurement remains the gold standard for the prediction of future fracture risk. Prospective studies show a doubling of fracture risk for every 1 standard deviation decrease in BMD. This predictive value is therefore at least as good as the use of blood pressure values to detect stroke risk [26].

However, axial DXA is not available to all primary or secondary care teams. pDXA measurement at the calcaneus is the second best predictor of hip fracture risk, after femoral neck BMD [30], and is as useful as lumbar spine BMD for predicting future vertebral fractures [31]. Calcaneal ultrasound can be used to predict hip fracture in middle-aged and elderly women [32,33]. Thus, even if axial DXA is unavailable, primary care teams can use clinical risk factors combined with other bone measurement technologies to identify those with high fracture risk. The current guidance, use, and limitations of pDXA, QUS, and axial DXA in selective case finding are discussed further in **Chapter 5**.

Hip fracture risk factor scores

Prediction of hip fracture risk is possible using Cummings' risk factors. These are shown in **Table 4.5**. Cummings et al. found that patients with five or more risk factors have a 25 times greater hip fracture risk than those with two or fewer risk factors. This risk factor score is useful for identifying groups of high-risk, frail, elderly women who can then be targeted with fall prevention programs,

Age >80 years	More than two cups of coffee per day
Fracture since the age of 50 years	Standing <4 hours per day
Maternal hip fracture	No walking for exercise
Poor/very poor health	Unable to rise from chair without using arms
Anticonvulsant treatment	
Long-acting benzodiazepine treatment	Previous hyperparathyroidism
Weight less than at age 25 years	Lowest quartile depth perception
Height at age 25 years >168 cm	Lowest quartile contrast sensitivity

Table 4.5 Cummings' hip fracture risk factors.

Direct referral from orthopedic service to osteoporosis service
GPs recommended to refer for GP Direct Access Densitometry
Direct referral for dual-energy X-ray absorptiometry from the accident and emergency department
Fracture Initiative Service with operational support nurses and trauma liaison nurses

Table 4.6 Options for selective case finding in patients with new fractures.
GP: general practitioner.

calcium, and/or vitamin D (or bisphosphonates if previous fragility fracture), where appropriate.

Opportunistic selective case finding

Fragility fracture at one site is a strong predictor of future fracture at the same and other sites, yet, unfortunately, many patients who fracture are not fully assessed and treated [3]. If strategies were in place to consistently diagnose and treat osteoporosis at the time of the first fragility fracture, much pain, suffering, and cost could be avoided.

In several centers in the UK, patients presenting with fragility fractures are identified on admission or when attending the fracture clinic. They are assessed for osteoporosis risk factors and either treated or, if the diagnosis of osteoporosis is uncertain and they are under age 75 years, a DXA scan is taken. If they have osteoporosis, bone-sparing therapy can be initiated.

Different models of selective case finding that can be applied to those who have sustained fractures are summarized in **Table 4.6**. Direct referral, either to the osteoporosis service from an orthopedic department or back to GPs for onward referral for DXA, if appropriate, may result in a significant delay in diagnosis; moreover, not all of those with fractures will be assessed, and direct GP access to DXA is not universally available. However, these strategies remain useful in centers without a Fracture Initiative Service. Fracture patients not identified at

In-patients	Out-patients
Fragility fracture patients identified on admission	Fragility fracture patients identified in fracture clinic
Investigations completed Patient details to database	Investigations completed Patient details to database
Osteoporosis ward round – decision on need for DXA and appropriate treatment in agreement with consultant	Patients seen by operational support nurse in clinic – decision on need for DXA and appropriate treatment in agreement with consultant
Operational support nurse provides education about the disease and treatment	Operational support nurse provides education about the disease and treatment
Investigation results and treatment recommendation recorded in assessment sheets – copy retained in notes and copy sent to general practitioner with discharge summary	Investigation results and treatment recommendation recorded in assessment sheets – copy retained in notes and copy sent to general practitioner with fracture clinic note
General practitioner and patient advice and support available by telephone from Osteoporosis Service	Patient attends general practitioner for treatment initiation; general practitioner and patient advice and support available by telephone from Osteoporosis Service
Ongoing audit of service	Ongoing audit of service

Table 4.7 Example of a fracture initiative care pathway. DXA: dual-energy X-ray absorptiometry.

this stage can be identified retrospectively as part of the 'search and rescue' recommendations for primary care, discussed below.

A Fracture Initiative Service was piloted in Glasgow, and is now in place in many centers around the UK. An example of a care pathway is shown in **Table 4.7**, but many different models are effective.

'Search and rescue' selective case finding
This is most applicable to primary care, where patient records are available for searching either by computer or manually. A variety of computer audits can be carried out, as shown in **Table 4.8**. As with any computer search, the ability to identify high-risk patients relies on good data entry. It is easiest to begin by tackling a group of high-risk patients who are easy to identify by computer search. Patients identified can then be 'rescued' by appropriate treatment to reduce their future fracture risk. A simple audit cycle is shown in **Figure 4.1**.

Organizational issues

Implementation of strategies in the primary care setting
Primary care physicians have to deal with all acute and chronic disease; therefore, concise guidance on implementing a selective case-finding strategy in

| Previous fragility fracture |
| Oral glucocorticoid therapy |
| Hysterectomy and oophorectomy before the age of 45 years |
| Frail, elderly patients who are housebound or in nursing or residential homes |

Table 4.8 Audits of high-risk patients.

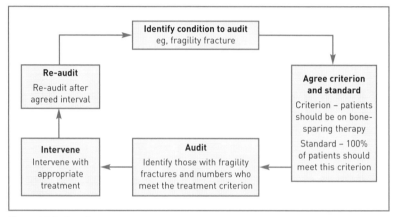

Figure 4.1 Audit cycle.

an individual practice or across a primary care organization will be useful. Information from other chapters of this book can be combined with the strategy information provided here to formulate a five-step management plan for use in primary care settings, as shown in **Figure 4.2**.

European Bone and Joint Health Strategies Project

This is a joint initiative between the Bone and Joint Decade, the European League against Rheumatism, the International Osteoporosis Foundation, and the European Federation of National Associations of Orthopedics and Traumatology, which aims to reduce the burden of bone and joint disorders within Europe. It is hoped that the project will result in the implementation of strategies across the European Union at local, regional, and national levels to reduce the impact of osteoporosis, osteoarthritis, rheumatoid arthritis, back pain, major limb trauma, and occupational and sports injuries.

The incidence, prevalence, and impact of osteoporosis have been quantified, in addition to the identification of risk factors and interventions suitable for use in those at risk of the disease, those with early disease, and those with advanced osteoporosis. Strategies and policies to reduce the burden of osteoporosis by building on existing service provision are being developed, together with

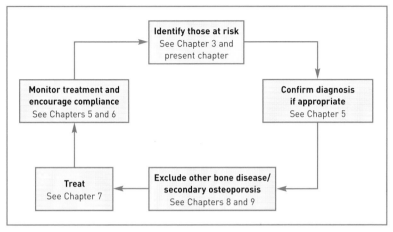

Figure 4.2 Example of a five-step management plan for use in primary care settings.

recommendations for how these can be implemented in differing healthcare environments. The project recognizes the importance of suitably motivational incentive schemes to encourage implementation, and recognizes that the difficulty lies not with the development of evidence-based guidelines, but with their implementation [34].

Conclusion

Osteoporosis has a lower profile than most chronic diseases. However, osteoporotic fractures are expensive to treat, and cause significant mortality, morbidity, and loss of independence; many are largely preventable with appropriate treatment. Previous fragility fracture, oral glucocorticoid use, other clinical risk factors, falls risk assessment, and clinical signs/symptoms can be used for selective case finding of those at highest risk of future fracture. These individuals can then be offered appropriate therapy to reduce their risk of subsequent fracture. Education and funding are vital in primary and secondary care to ensure that teams have the tools and resources needed to implement a selective case-finding strategy, and to treat those identified as being at highest risk.

Targeting the entire population with advice about lifestyle modifications to optimize PBM and prevent loss later in life, in a 'cradle to the grave' approach, fits synergistically with the advice offered for the prevention of other chronic diseases, and may result in small beneficial improvements in BMD across the population. However, with limited resources, selective case-finding and targeting treatment to those at highest risk of fractures is more cost-effective and must take priority.

References

1. World Health Organization. Assessment of fracture risk and its application to screening for postmenopausal osteoporosis. *WHO Technical Report Series.* Geneva: WHO, 1994.

2. Freemantle N. Screening for osteoporosis to prevent fracture. *Effective Health Care Bulletin*;1. Leeds: School of Public Health, 1992.

3. Cooper C, Melton LJ III. Vertebral fractures: how large is the silent epidemic? *BMJ* 1992;304:793–4.

4. Heaney RP, Abrams S, Dawson-Hughes B, et al. Peak bone mass. *Osteoporos Int* 2000;11:985–1009.

5. Bassey E. Exercise for improving bone mineral density: the benefits of weight training. *Osteoporos Rev* 2001;9:11–13.

6. Lohman T, Going S, Pamenter R, et al. Effects of resistance training on regional and total bone mineral density in premenopausal women: a randomized prospective study. *J Bone Miner Res* 1995;10:1015–24.

7. Feder G, Cryer C, Donovan S, et al. Guidelines for the prevention of falls in people over 65. *BMJ* 2000;321:1007–11.

8. Pereira MA, Kriska AM, Day RD, et al. A randomised walking trial in post-menopausal women: Effects on physical activity and health 10 years later. *Arch Intern Med* 1998;158:1695–701.

9. Province MA, Hadley EC, Hornbrook MC, et al. The effects of exercise on falls in elderly patients. A preplanned meta-analysis of the FICSIT trials. *JAMA* 1995;273:1341–7.

10. Campbell AJ, Robertson MC, Gardner MM, et al. Randomized controlled trial of a general practice programme of home based exercise to prevent falls in elderly women. *BMJ* 1997;315:1065–9.

11. Gregory J, Lowe C Bates C, et al. National Diet and Nutrition Survey: young people aged 4 to 18 years. Volume 1: *Report of the Diet and Nutrition Survey.* London: The Stationery Office, 2000.

12. Finch S, Doyle W, Lowe C, et al. National Diet and Nutrition Survey: people aged 65 years or over. Volume 1: *Report of the Diet and Nutrition Survey.* London: The Stationery Office, 1998.

13. New SA, Robins SP, Campbell MK, et al. Dietary influences on bone mass and bone metabolism: further evidence of a positive link between fruit and vegetable consumption and bone health? *Am J Clin Nutr* 2000;71:142–51.

14. Tucker KL, Hannan MT, Chen H. Potassium, magnesium, and fruit and vegetable intakes are associated with greater bone mineral density in elderly men and women. *Am J Clin Nutr* 1999;69:727–36.

15. Booth SL, Tucker KL, Chen H, et al. Dietary vitamin K intakes are associated with hip fracture but not with bone mineral density in elderly men and women. *Am J Clin Nutr* 2000;71:1201–8.

16. Hannan MT, Tucker KL, Dawson-Hughes B, et al. Effect of dietary protein on bone loss in elderly men and women. The Framingham Study. *J Bone Miner Res* 2000;15:2504–12.

17. Avenell A, Handoll HHG. Nutritional supplementation for hip fracture aftercare in the elderly. Oxford: Cochrane Library, 2000.

18. Barrett-Connor E, Chang JC, Edelstein SL. Coffee-associated osteoporosis offset by daily milk consumption. The Rancho Bernardo Study. *JAMA* 1994;271:280–3.

19. Kiel DP, Felson DT, Hannan MT, et al. Caffeine and the risk of hip fracture: the Framingham Study. *Am J Epidemiol* 1990;132:675–84.

20. Harris SS, Dawson-Hughes B. Caffeine and bone loss in healthy menopausal women. *Am J Clin Nutr* 1994;60:573–8

21. Baron JA, Farahmand BY, Weiderpass E, et al. Cigarette smoking, alcohol consumption and risk of hip fracture in women. *Arch Intern Med* 2001;161:983–8.

22. Hoidrup S, Gronbaek M, Gottschau A, et al. Alcohol intake, beverage preference, and risk of hip fracture in men and women. *Am J Epidemiol* 1999;149:993–1001.

23. Law MR, Hackshaw AK. A meta-analysis of cigarette smoking, bone mineral density and risk of hip fracture: recognition of a major effect. *BMJ* 1997;315:841–6.

24. Johnston CC Jr, Miller JZ, Slemenda CW, et al. Calcium supplementation and increases in bone mineral density in children. *N Engl J Med* 1992;327:82–7.

25. Bonjour JP, Carrie AL, Ferrari S, et al. Calcium-enriched foods and bone mass growth in prepubertal girls: a randomized double-blind placebo controlled trial. *J Clin Invest* 1997;99:1287–94.

26. Guideline development group for the Royal College of Physicians. *Osteoporosis: Clinical Guidelines for Prevention and Treatment.* London: Royal College of Physicians, 1999.

27. Kanis JA, Johnell O, Oden A, et al. Ten year risk of osteoporotic fracture and the effect of risk factors on screening strategy. *Bone* 2002;30:251–8.

28. Melton LJ III. Epidemiology of vertebral fractures in women. *Am J Epidemiol* 1989;129:1000–11.

29. Cummings SR, Black DM, Nevitt MC, et al. The Study of Osteoporotic Fractures Research Group. Bone density at various sites for prediction of hip fractures. *Lancet* 1993;341:72–5.

30. Marshall D, Johnell O, Wedel H. Meta-analysis of how well measures of bone density predict occurrence of osteoporotic fractures. *BMJ* 1996;312:1254–9.

31. Hans D, Dargent-Molina P, Schott AM, et al. Ultrasonographic heel measurements to predict hip fractures in elderly women: the EPIDOS study. *Lancet* 1996;348:511–14.

32. Thompson PW, Taylor J, Oliver R, et al. Quantitative ultrasound of the heel predicts wrist and osteoporosis related fractures in women aged 45–75. *J Clin Densitom* 1998;3:219–25.

33. Cummings SR, Nevitt MC, Browner WS, et al. Risk factors for hip fracture in white women. Study of Osteoporotic Fractures Research Group. *N Engl J Med* 1995;332:767–73.

34. The European Bone and Joint Health Strategies Project. European Action Towards Better Musculoskeletal Health. Available from: www.europa.eu.int. ISBN-91-975284-0-4.

5

The Radiologic Diagnosis of Osteoporosis

Glen Blake and Ignac Fogelman

Introduction

The introduction of the first dual-energy X-ray absorptiometry (DXA) scanning systems in the late 1980s marked the beginning of a period of rapid growth in the clinical applications of bone densitometry [1]. Today, scans to measure bone mineral density (BMD) are seen as having an essential role in the evaluation of patients at risk of osteoporosis [2,3]. Growing awareness of the impact of osteoporosis on the elderly population [4], the consequent costs of healthcare [5,6], and the development of new treatments to prevent fractures [7–10] have led to rapid growth in the demand for bone densitometry services.

With continued improvements in technology, scan times have decreased from around 10 minutes for the first generation DXA systems to only a few seconds today. Alongside conventional densitometry of the spine and hip, a variety of different types of equipment are now available for making measurements in the peripheral skeleton. With its advantages of high precision, short scan times, low radiation dose, and stable calibration, DXA has proved well suited to meet the need for patient measurement equipment to assist in the diagnosis of osteoporosis and aid decisions about treatment.

The radiologic definition of osteoporosis

In the early 1990s, a consensus meeting defined osteoporosis as "a systemic skeletal disease characterized by low bone mass and microarchitectural deterioration of bone tissue, with a consequent increase in bone fragility and susceptibility to fracture" [11]. It should be noted that this definition does not require an individual to have sustained a fracture before a diagnosis of osteoporosis is made, but introduces the concept of low bone mass and its relationship to increased fracture risk. While it could be argued that it is wrong to define a disease on the basis of what is essentially a risk factor (ie, low BMD), there is nevertheless some logic to this, as fractures tend to occur late in the disease process when skeletal integrity is already

Terminology	T-score definition
Normal	T ≥−1.0
Osteopenia	−2.5 < T <−1.0
Osteoporosis	T ≤−2.5
Established osteoporosis	T ≤−2.5 in the presence of one or more fragility fractures

Table 5.1 The World Health Organization recommendations for the definitions of osteoporosis and osteopenia.

severely compromised. It is therefore desirable to identify those individuals at high risk with a view to instituting appropriate treatment.

Today, there is general agreement that BMD measurements are the most effective way of identifying those patients most at risk of fracture. Indeed, the widespread availability of DXA systems has led to a working definition of osteoporosis based on BMD. In 1994, a World Health Organization (WHO) report recommended a clinical definition of osteoporosis based on a BMD measurement of the spine, hip, or forearm, expressed in standard deviation (SD) units called T-scores [12]. A patient's T-score is calculated by taking the difference between the measured BMD and the mean BMD of healthy young adults matched for gender and ethnic group, and expressing the difference relative to the SD of the young adult population:

$$\text{T-score} = \frac{\text{Measured BMD} - \text{Young adult mean BMD}}{\text{Young adult SD}}$$

A T-score indicates the difference between the patient's measured BMD and the ideal peak bone mass achieved by a young adult [13]. A negative T-score means that either the patient failed to achieve the optimum peak bone mass or subsequently lost bone mass due to the effects of aging or disease. The WHO report classifies a patient as having osteoporosis if their T-score is ≤−2.5 at the spine, hip, or forearm (**Table 5.1**).

The WHO study also proposed an intermediate state, referred to as osteopenia, defined by a T-score between −2.5 and −1. A T-score ≥−1 was regarded as normal. A fourth state of 'established osteoporosis' was also proposed, denoting osteoporosis as defined above, but in the presence of one or more documented fragility fractures. The WHO report definitions of osteoporosis, osteopenia, and normal BMD are intended to identify patients with high, intermediate, and low risk of fracture, respectively. However, an important limitation of these definitions is that they apply only to DXA measurements at the sites specified and cannot automatically be applied to other sites in the skeleton or to alternative measurement techniques [14].

The rationale for the WHO definition of osteoporosis is that it describes the disease in around 30% of white postmenopausal women [3]. This figure was chosen because it approximates to the lifetime risk of fracture for a 50-year-old white woman [12]. In comparison, it can be argued that the WHO definition of osteopenia captures too high a percentage of women to be clinically useful, and nowadays this term is used less often, particularly in the context of therapeutic decision making.

In contrast, the WHO definition of osteoporosis has had a major influence on clinical practice, to the extent that the question: 'Does this patient have osteoporosis?' will be answered using T-scores. Alongside the T-score, another useful way to express BMD measurements is using Z-scores. Like the T-score, the Z-score is expressed in units of the population SD. However, instead of comparing the patient's BMD with the young adult mean, it is compared with the mean for a healthy subject matched for age, gender, and ethnic origin:

$$\text{Z-score} = \frac{\text{Measured BMD} - \text{Age-matched mean BMD}}{\text{Age-matched SD}}$$

Although Z-scores cannot be used to diagnose osteoporosis, they nevertheless remain a useful concept because they express a patient's risk of sustaining an osteoporotic fracture relative to their peers. Every 1 SD reduction in BMD equates to an approximate 2-fold increase in the likelihood of fracture [15]. It follows that patients with a Z-score of <-1 are at a substantially increased risk of fracture compared with their peers.

Dual-energy X-ray absorptiometry

DXA is one of several techniques available for the noninvasive radiologic assessment of the skeleton (**Table 5.2**). This chapter will concentrate on the use of DXA measurements at sites in the central skeleton (spine and hip) and the peripheral skeleton (forearm, hand, and heel), since these are the most widely used types of measurement. The DXA technique used for making measurements of the peripheral skeleton is often referred to as peripheral (p)DXA. This chapter will also briefly review some alternative techniques, such as quantitative computed tomography (QCT) [16], quantitative ultrasound (QUS) [17], radiographic absorptiometry (RA) [18], and radiogrammetry [19].

DXA bone density measurements of the central skeleton

DXA equipment for the assessment of the central skeleton is used for BMD measurements of the spine and hip (**Figures 5.1–5.3**). These are usually regarded as the sites of most clinical importance because they are frequent sites of fractures that cause substantial impairment of quality of life, morbidity, and mortality. A measurement of hip BMD has been shown to be the most reliable way of evaluating the risk of hip fracture [15,20]. Also, because of the metabolically active trabecular bone in the vertebral bodies, the spine is

Technique	Region of interest	Units reported	Precision (%CV)	Effective dose (μSv)
Central skeleton				
DXA	PA spine	BMD (g/cm²)	1%	1–10
	Proximal femur		1–2%	1–10
	Total body		1%	3
QCT	Spine	BMD (g/cm³)	3%	50–500
Peripheral skeleton				
pDXA	Forearm	BMD (g/cm²)	1–2%	0.1
	Calcaneus		1–2%	0.1
pQCT	Forearm	BMD (g/cm²)	1–2%	0.3
RA and radiogrammetry	Phalanx	BMD (g/cm²)	1–2%	10
QUS	Calcaneus	BUA (dB/MHz)	2–5%	None
	Calcaneus	SOS (m/s)	0.1–1%	None
	Tibia	SOS (m/s)	1–2%	None
	Multi-site	SOS (m/s)	1–2%	None

Table 5.2 Characteristics of different bone densitometry techniques. BMD: bone mineral density; BUA: broadband ultrasonic attenuation; CV: coefficient of variation; DXA: dual-energy X-ray absorptiometry; PA: posteroanterior; pDXA: peripheral dual-energy X-ray absorptiometry; pQCT: peripheral quantitative computed tomography; QCT: quantitative computed tomography; QUS: quantitative ultrasound; RA: radiographic absorptiometry; SOS: speed of sound.

regarded as the optimum site for monitoring the response to treatment [21]. The radiation dose is low, comparable with the average daily dose from natural background radiation [22]. DXA scanning of the central skeleton has become the most widely used bone densitometry technique because of its ability to measure spine and hip BMD with good precision, and to identify patients with osteoporosis on the basis of the WHO T-score definition.

Total body BMD can also be studied with this type of equipment (**Figure 5.4**). These studies are of interest because they show changes across the whole skeleton, including the skull, arms, ribs, thoracic and lumbar spine, pelvis, and legs. Such measurements are useful in trials of new treatments for osteoporosis because they address the issue of whether BMD gains at some sites are at the expense of losses elsewhere in the skeleton [23]. Total body DXA scans may also be used in body composition studies to measure whole body fat and lean mass.

A fourth type of scan can be performed on most spine and hip DXA systems, and comprises study of the distal forearm (**Figure 5.5**). This scan mode can be useful as an alternative site in patients in whom the hip or spine cannot be measured, eg, in patients with metal implants or bilateral hip prostheses.

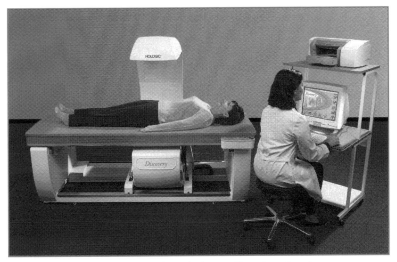

Figure 5.1 The Horologic Discovery fan-beam dual-energy X-ray absorptiometry scanner. Densitometers such as this are most frequently used for measuring spine and hip bone mineral density (BMD), but can also be used for total body and forearm BMD studies.

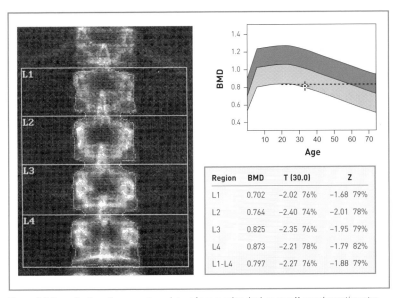

Region	BMD	T (30.0)		Z	
L1	0.702	−2.02	76%	−1.68	79%
L2	0.764	−2.40	74%	−2.01	78%
L3	0.825	−2.35	76%	−1.95	79%
L4	0.873	−2.21	78%	−1.79	82%
L1-L4	0.797	−2.27	76%	−1.88	79%

Figure 5.2 Reproduction of a computer printout from a spine dual-energy X-ray absorptiometry scan. The printout shows: **(left)** scan image of the lumbar spine; **(top right)** patient's age and bone mineral density (BMD) plotted with respect to the reference range; **(bottom right)** BMD figures for individual vertebrae and total spine (L1–L4), together with interpretation in terms of T-scores and Z-scores.

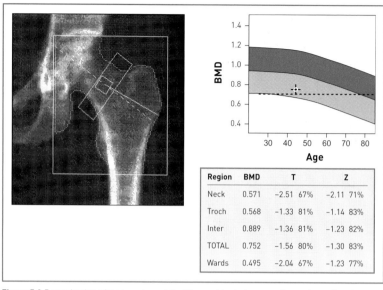

Figure 5.3 Reproduction of a computer printout from a hip dual-energy X-ray absorptiometry scan. The printout shows: **(left)** scan image of the hip; **(top right)** patient's age and bone mineral density (BMD) for the total hip region of interest (ROI) plotted with respect to the National Health and Nutrition Examination Survey (NHANES) III reference range [61]; **(bottom right)** BMD figures for five different ROIs in the hip (femoral neck, greater trochanter, intertrochanteric, total hip, and Ward's triangle), together with interpretation in terms of T-scores and Z-scores using the NHANES III reference range.

Region	Area (cm²)	BMC (gms)	BMD (gms/cm²)
L Arm	153.80	96.90	0.630
R Arm	171.06	109.09	0.638
L Ribs	111.43	63.54	0.638
R Ribs	121.63	71.63	0.589
T Spine	122.02	89.03	0.730
L Spine	43.55	34.80	0.799
Pelvis	172.63	161.40	0.935
L Leg	300.54	302.95	1.008
R Leg	295.04	298.36	1.011
Sub Tot	1491.69	1227.70	0.823
Head	209.12	444.51	2.126
TOTAL	17000.81	1672.21	0.983

Figure 5.4 Reproduction of a computer printout from a total body dual-energy X-ray absorptiometry scan. The printout shows: **(left)** scan image of the total body; **(right)** bone mineral density (BMD) figures for the total body and subregions. BMC: bone mineral content.

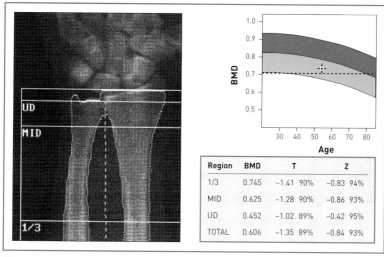

Region	BMD	T		Z	
1/3	0.745	−1.41	90%	−0.83	94%
MID	0.625	−1.28	90%	−0.86	93%
UD	0.452	−1.02	89%	−0.42	95%
TOTAL	0.606	−1.35	89%	−0.84	93%

Figure 5.5 Reproduction of a computer printout from a forearm dual-energy X-ray absorptiometry scan. The printout shows: **(left)** scan image of the distal forearm; **(top right)** patient's age and bone mineral density (BMD) for the one-third region of interest (ROI) plotted with respect to the reference range; **(bottom right)** BMD figures for four different ROIs in the forearm (ultradistal, mid-, one-third, and total forearm), together with interpretation in terms of T-scores and Z-scores.

The fundamental principle behind DXA is the measurement of the transmission of X-rays of two different photon energies through the body. Because of the dependence of transmission attenuation on atomic number and photon energy, measurement of the transmission at two energies enables the densities of two different types of tissue to be inferred. In DXA scanning, the two tissues are taken to be bone mineral (hydroxyapatite) and soft tissue. Because DXA measurements are based on a two-dimensional projection image and not a three-dimensional tomographic image, the bone density figures obtained are not true physical densities (ie, mass per unit volume in units of g/cm³), but so called 'areal' densities, representing the mass per unit projected area in units of g/cm².

DXA measurements are made by resolving the transmission factors at two different photon energies into the equivalent areal densities of two well-defined types of tissue. However, soft-tissue has a variable fat and lean composition, and the attenuation of X-ray photons by fat is different to that of lean tissue. Differences in the soft tissue composition in the path of the X-ray beam through bone compared with the adjacent soft tissue will cause errors in BMD measurements. These have been examined in a number of studies. Svendsen et al. reported a cadaver study that examined the random accuracy errors of BMD measurements in the forearm, spine, and hip caused by the effects of fat inhomogeneity [24]. The root mean square errors were reported to be 3% for forearm, 5% for spine, and 6% for hip BMD measurements.

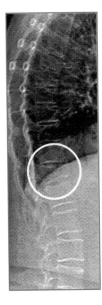

Figure 5.6 Lateral vertebral assessment image of the lumbar and thoracic spine. Images such as this obtained using dual-energy X-ray absorptiometry systems can be evaluated for evidence of vertebral fractures.

The first generation of DXA scanners used a pinhole collimator that produced a pencil beam coupled to a single scintillation detector in the scanning arm. A spine or hip study with a pencil beam system entailed a two-dimensional raster scan that took 5–10 minutes to complete. Subsequently, more advanced systems were introduced that used a slit collimator to generate a fan beam coupled to a linear array of solid state detectors. Image resolution was improved, and because the scanning arm moved in only one direction, scan times were shortened to 10–30 seconds. In the latest generation DXA systems, two-dimensional detector arrays developed for digital radiography systems have been used to develop a cone-beam system in which image acquisition takes only 1–2 seconds [25].

Identification of vertebral fractures

Clinical trials of new treatments for osteoporosis conducted during the 1990s emphasized the importance of a prevalent vertebral fracture as a risk factor for future fracture. Studies suggest that, independently of BMD, patients with a prevalent vertebral fracture are at substantially greater risk of further fracture than patients without a prevalent fracture [26]. Conventionally, the diagnosis of vertebral fracture is made from lateral X-ray films of the lumbar and thoracic spine [27]. However, the new generation of fan-beam and cone-beam DXA systems are designed to acquire fast, high-resolution lateral images of the spine that may provide equivalent information (**Figure 5.6**).

Advantages of lateral vertebral imaging using DXA equipment include the low radiation dose compared with X-ray films, and the ability to combine an assessment for vertebral fracture and a BMD measurement at a single patient

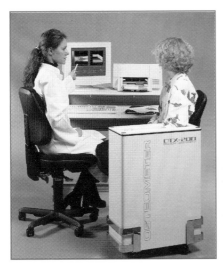

Figure 5.7 The Osteometer DTX-200 forearm dual-energy X-ray absorptiometry (DXA) scanner. Peripheral DXA systems are smaller and cheaper than spine and hip DXA systems, such as that shown in **Figure 5.1**. Reproduced with permission from Osteometer MediTech, Inc.

visit [28]. Initial studies have shown good agreement between DXA imaging and conventional radiographs, despite the rather poorer spatial resolution of the DXA images [29].

DXA bone density measurements of the peripheral skeleton

Despite the widespread popularity of spine and hip DXA, there is continuing interest in new pDXA devices for assessing sites in the peripheral skeleton.

The first densitometers were forearm scanners that used the technique of single-photon absorptiometry based on a radionuclide source [30]. Follow-up of patients after single photon absorptiometry studies has shown that forearm bone density measurements can predict fracture risk over 25 years [31]. In recent years, the technology has been updated by replacing the radionuclide source with a low voltage X-ray tube and using the principles of DXA to perform BMD scans of the distal forearm (**Figure 5.7**). Similar devices are used to scan the heel and the hand. The advantages of pDXA systems include their small size, relatively low cost, and extremely low radiation dose [32].

pDXA has significant advantages when selecting equipment suitable for use in primary care. However, epidemiologic studies show that the discriminatory ability of peripheral BMD measurements to predict hip fractures is somewhat poorer than when hip BMD measurements are used [15,20]. Also, these types of measurement are less suitable than spine BMD for follow-up scans [33]. Finally, despite the fact that the radiation dose is extremely low, peripheral X-ray devices are subject to government regulatory requirements controlling the use of radiographic equipment, including the training of technologists and physicians in the principles of radiation safety.

Alternative techniques for skeletal assessment

Quantitative computed tomography

The alternative technique of QCT [16] has the advantage that it measures the true physical density (g/cm^3) compared with the two-dimensional areal density that is measured by DXA. It therefore avoids the errors associated with DXA due to variations in bone size. QCT is usually applied to measure the trabecular bone in the vertebral bodies. The measurement can be performed on any clinical computed tomography (CT) scanner, provided that the patient is scanned with an external reference phantom to calibrate the CT numbers to equivalent bone values. Most CT manufacturers provide a software package to automate the placement of the regions of interest (ROI) within the vertebral bodies. Patient radiation dose is much lower than for standard CT scans, provided that the examination is performed correctly [34].

The advantage of spinal QCT is the high responsiveness of the vertebral trabecular bone to aging and disease [35]. The principal disadvantage is the relative cost of the equipment. Just as pDXA devices offer a smaller, cheaper means of performing DXA studies at sites in the peripheral skeleton, peripheral (p)QCT scanners are miniaturized CT devices for taking BMD measurements in the forearm or tibia. Since the radiation dose is very low and true density is measured (unaffected by bone size), pQCT devices are particularly suitable for investigations in children.

Radiographic absorptiometry and radiogrammetry

RA is a technique that was developed many years ago for assessing BMD in the hand, but has recently attracted renewed interest [18]. A standard radiograph of the hand is obtained with a small aluminum wedge for calibration (**Figure 5.8a**). The film is then scanned into a personal computer and the image processed to measure BMD (**Figure 5.8b**).

In the similar technique of radiogrammetry, the aluminum wedge is dispensed with and measurements of the periosteal and intraluminal diameters of the metacarpals on the X-ray image are used to estimate BMD [19]. The advantage of these techniques is their potential for general use on the basis of the widespread availability of conventional film radiography.

Quantitative ultrasound

QUS is a new technique for measuring the peripheral skeleton and has raised considerable interest in recent years [17]. There is a wide variety of equipment available, with most devices using the heel as the measurement site [36]. The calcaneus is chosen because it encompasses a large volume of trabecular bone between relatively flat faces, and is readily accessible for transmission measurements.

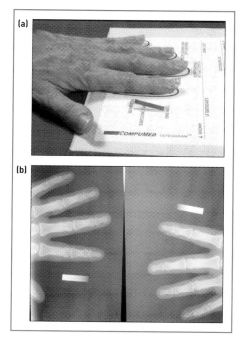

Figure 5.8 (a) In radiographic absorptiometry, an X-ray film of the hand is calibrated with a small aluminum wedge. **(b)** The resulting film can be digitized to measure bone mineral density in the phalanges.

The physical measurements made are usually a measure of the attenuation of the ultrasound signal through the bone, referred to as broadband ultrasonic attenuation (BUA), and the speed of sound (SOS) through the heel. The values of both BUA and SOS are reduced in patients with osteoporosis. With most early-generation QUS devices, the patient's foot was placed in a water bath to couple the ultrasound signal to the heel. However, newer devices are dry contact systems in which rubber pads covered with ultrasound gel are pressed against the patient's heel (**Figure 5.9**).

A major attraction of bone ultrasound devices is that they do not use ionizing radiation, and therefore avoid the regulatory requirements for X-ray systems mentioned above. Also, the instrumentation is relatively inexpensive, and several devices, especially among the dry systems, are designed to be portable. Therefore, ultrasound could be more widely used than conventional DXA scanners, which are largely restricted to hospital-based osteoporosis clinics. The case for QUS is strengthened by evidence from several large prospective studies, confirming that QUS measurements predict hip fracture risk as effectively as DXA [37–39].

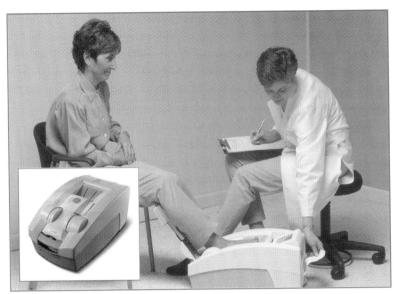

Figure 5.9 The GE Achilles Insight ultrasonometer used for performing measurements in the heel. Devices such as this measure broadband ultrasonic attenuation and speed of sound in the calcaneus. Reproduced with permission from GE Healthcare.

The clinical use of bone densitometry measurements

In general, bone densitometry measurements have three different roles in the investigation and treatment of osteoporosis. Firstly, they are used to diagnose osteoporosis based on the WHO definition of a T-score less than or equal to –2.5 at the spine, hip, or forearm [12]. As emphasized previously, this definition applies only to white women, and only to DXA measurements at the sites specified [14]. Although it may be possible in the future to define equivalent thresholds applicable to the other types of measurement, there is presently no consensus on how this should be done [40,41].

The second use of bone densitometry studies is to assess a patient's risk of a fragility fracture. The most convincing method of demonstrating the ability of scans to predict fracture risk is through epidemiologic studies [15,20]. Based on present knowledge, the most effective use of DXA equipment is to use hip BMD scans to predict hip fracture risk [42].

The third use of bone densitometry is in longitudinal studies to assess a patient's response to treatment [21]. These studies are of two types:

- research studies made during trials of new treatments for osteoporosis
- monitoring the response of individual patients commencing treatment

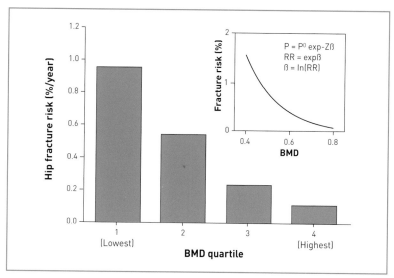

The equations shown in the inset graph:

$$P = P^0 \exp{-Z\beta}$$
$$RR = \exp\beta$$
$$\beta = \ln(RR)$$

Figure 5.10 Incidence of hip fracture by bone mineral density (BMD) quartile for femoral neck BMD. Data are taken from the Study of Osteoporotic Fractures (SOF) [20]. Data from fracture studies such as SOF are fitted using a gradient-of-risk model, in which fracture risk varies exponentially with Z-score. Results are given in terms of the relative risk (RR), the increased risk of fracture for each unit decrease in Z-score.

The use of DXA scanning in clinical trials has made an important contribution to the evaluation of new treatments for osteoporosis [7–10,43–49].

Underlying such studies is an assumption that an increase in BMD is indicative of a decrease in fracture risk, and it is important that this is verified in fracture prevention studies [7–10,45–48]. The second type of longitudinal study, the monitoring of individual patients, is more controversial [50]. It is widely believed that follow-up scans in patients commencing treatment encourage them to continue with their medication, and are also useful in identifying nonresponders who may benefit from a different treatment regimen. How effective follow-up studies are in either of these roles is a matter of current debate. The remainder of this chapter will examine each of these roles in turn.

The assessment of fracture risk

Which type of measurement is best?

Although the most frequent reason for performing a BMD scan is to make the diagnosis of osteoporosis, fundamental to this is the ability of scans to assess fracture risk. The comparison of different types of bone densitometry equipment in predicting fracture risk is therefore essential when choosing the most effective type of measurement. The most reliable approach to this issue is through

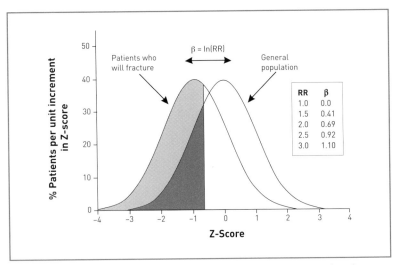

Figure 5.11 Gaussian curves representing the distribution of bone mineral density (BMD) values in a fracture population compared with the age-matched general population. The curve representing the fracture population has the same standard deviation as the curve representing the general population, but is offset to lower BMD values by a Z-score difference of $\Delta Z = \ln(RR)$ [51].

prospective epidemiologic studies [15]. **Figure 5.10** illustrates how data from such a study are analyzed to quantify the relationship between a bone densitometry measurement and the associated fracture risk. When the baseline BMD values are used to divide patients into quartiles, an approximately exponential relationship between fracture risk and BMD is found. To describe this relationship, the BMD measurements are first converted into Z-score values. Results from the fracture study are then expressed as the increased risk of fracture for each unit decrease in Z-score, an index referred to as the relative risk (RR) (**Figure 5.10**, inset).

For subjects taken from the general population, the distribution of Z-score values approximates to a Gaussian curve (**Figure 5.11**). The distribution of Z-score values for the group of patients who will at some future date sustain a low-trauma fracture is found by multiplying the distribution curve representing the general population by the exponential fracture risk curve. When this is done, the Z-score distribution of the fracture population is found to be a curve similar to that describing the general population, but with its peak offset to the left by an amount $\Delta Z = \ln(RR)$ (**Figure 5.11**) [51].

The area under each of the two curves up to some chosen threshold can be evaluated to estimate the percentage of patients in the two populations with BMD values below the threshold. As the threshold is varied, and the percentages plotted against each other, we obtain a receiver operating characteristic curve

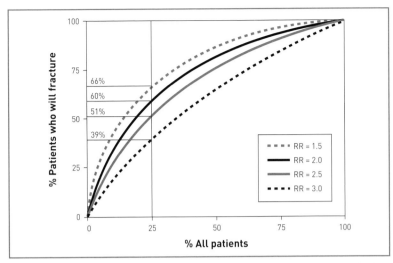

Figure 5.12 Plot of the receiver operating characteristic (ROC) curves obtained by integrating the two Gaussian curves in **Figure 5.11** for different values of relative risk (RR). The ROC curve shows the percentage of subjects in the fracture group who fall below any chosen bone mineral density (BMD) threshold plotted against the percentage of subjects in the general population who fall below the same threshold. It therefore shows the true positive fraction (those patients who sustain a fracture and were correctly identified as being at risk) plotted against the false positive fraction (those patients identified as being at risk but who never actually have a fracture). The larger the value of RR, the more effective the BMD measurements are at discriminating the patients at risk of fracture. For example, if patients in the lowest quartile of BMD are identified for treatment, then for RR values of 1.5, 2.0, 2.5, and 3.0 this group will include 39%, 51%, 60%, and 66%, respectively, of all patients who will suffer a fracture.

(**Figure 5.12**) [52] in which the true positive fraction (those patients who will later sustain a low-trauma fracture and were correctly identified to be at risk by the BMD measurement) is shown plotted against the false positive fraction (those patients identified as being at risk, but who never fracture). **Figure 5.12** is fundamental to understanding the clinical utility of any type of bone densitometry measurement used to identify and treat patients at risk of fracture [51]. It shows that the larger the RR value, the better the discrimination of the measurements in identifying those patients likely to sustain fractures.

It is clear from **Figure 5.12** that RR values derived from fracture studies provide key data for assessing the relative merits of different types of measurement. One of the largest of these studies, the Study of Osteoporotic Fractures (SOF), involved more than 9,000 women aged ≥65 years, recruited in four regions of the USA [20,53,54]. The most recent SOF data have provided highly statistically significant evidence that if the clinical aim is to prevent hip fractures, then femur BMD is the best measurement to use (**Figure 5.13**) [42].

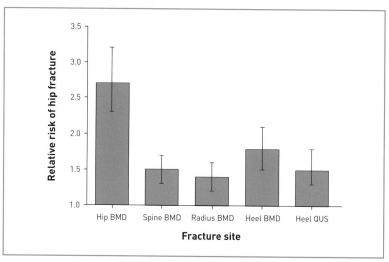

Figure 5.13 Relative risk values for 5-year hip fracture incidence for bone mineral density (BMD) measurements of the femoral neck, lumbar spine, forearm, and heel, and quantitative ultrasound measurements (QUS) of the heel. Data from Black et al [42].

For a wider view that includes other fracture sites, a meta-analysis of fracture studies is required. Marshall et al. published such an analysis, and their collated RR figures for the prediction of different types of fracture from BMD measurements at different skeletal sites are shown in **Figure 5.14** [15]. These data are widely taken as showing that fracture risk at a given skeletal site is best predicted by a BMD measurement at that site. Interestingly, when assessed by the ability to predict fractures occurring at any site, RR figures for BMD measurements at central and peripheral sites are closely comparable. This view is supported by the early results of the National Osteoporosis Risk Assessment study [55]. These showed RR values of around 1.5 for the prediction of any type of fracture by measurements on four different types of peripheral device [56].

What happens if different techniques disagree?

Given the range of different types of equipment, there is cause for concern about the potential for conflicting findings between different techniques. If two techniques correlate perfectly ($r = 1.0$), they will identify exactly the same patients as being at risk. However, in practice, different types of measurement often correlate poorly, with $r \approx 0.6$–0.7 between BMD results from different sites [35], and $r \approx 0.4$–0.5 between QUS and BMD results [57,58]. This raises the question of whether clinicians should be concerned that, due to these imperfect correlations, different patients may be selected for treatment on the basis of different types of measurement.

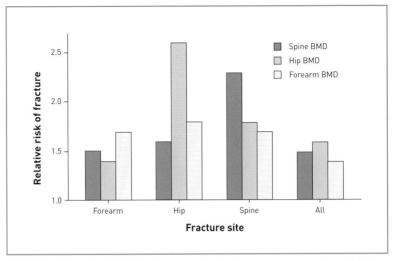

Figure 5.14 Relative risk values for fractures at different skeletal sites for bone mineral density (BMD) measurements in the spine, hip, and forearm. Data from Marshall et al [15].

These issues can be examined by generalizing the single variable Gaussian model shown in **Figure 5.11** to include scatter plots of two variables – eg, femur BMD versus QUS. Suppose that the correlation coefficient between the two measurements is $r = 0.5$. If a clinician were to treat patients in the lowest quartile of the age-matched population for both modalities, 60% of future fracture patients would be treated on the basis of a femur BMD measurement (RR = 2.5) compared with 51% on the basis of a QUS measurement (RR = 2.0). By extending the Gaussian model to a scatter plot of two variables, it can be estimated that 39% of future fracture patients would be identified by both techniques, while 28% of cases would be missed by both modalities (**Figure 5.15**).

This example is instructive because it emphasizes how the lack of agreement between techniques arises: different devices are selecting different groups from the total pool of patients who will sustain a fracture. In this instance, femur BMD is the better measurement because it identifies a larger percentage of future fracture cases.

It is clear that BMD studies provide a measure of fracture risk that is analogous to assessment of blood pressure with regard to the risk of stroke, or measurement of cholesterol with regard to the risk of ischemic heart disease [15]. It is important to distinguish the concepts of risk as applied to an individual and to a population. Although BMD is an important risk factor for fracture, fracture events are nevertheless multifactorial and depend upon other factors (eg, accidents and the propensity to fall). While BMD measurements are well suited to the study of populations, they are less good at identifying specific

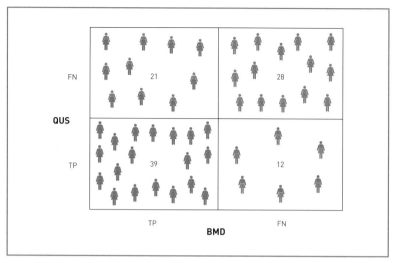

Figure 5.15 Comparison of the agreement between the treatment decisions based on femoral neck bone mineral density (BMD; relative risk [RR] = 2.5) and a quantitative ultrasound (QUS) measurement (RR = 2.0) for 100 future fracture patients. It is assumed that the correlation coefficient between the BMD and QUS measurements is $r = 0.5$, and that patients are recommended for treatment if they are in the lowest quartile of the measurements. On this basis, 60% of patients would have true positive (TP) BMD scans compared with 51% having TP QUS results. Also, 39% of patients would have TP scans by both techniques, and 28% of cases would have false negative scans (FN) by both modalities. The figure emphasizes that different types of measurement select different groups of individuals from the total pool of patients who will eventually sustain a fracture.

individuals who will later sustain a fracture. Since fracture risk varies exponentially with BMD, there will always be an overlap between measurements in fracture and nonfracture patients, and absolute discrimination between these groups is not possible using any type of BMD measurement (see **Figure 5.11**).

Making the diagnosis of osteoporosis

Which reference range to use?

If treatment of patients is based on BMD measurements expressed in T-scores, then any errors in the mean BMD or population SD of the reference group could have a significant influence on clinical decisions. The majority of centers that offer a scanning service use reference ranges provided by the equipment manufacturers; issues over the accuracy of these ranges have caused controversy in the past [59]. This continues to be a problematic area in view of the large number of new devices being introduced. However, the problem was resolved for femur DXA after a report by the International Committee for Standards in Bone Measurement (ICSBM) [60], which recommended that hip BMD

History of fracture after age 40 years
History of hip, wrist, or vertebral fracture in a first-degree relative
Being in lowest quartile for body weight (≤57.8 kg [127 lb])
Current cigarette smoking habit

Table 5.3 Risk factors for osteoporosis, additional to age and bone mineral density, incorporated in the National Osteoporosis Foundation guidelines for therapeutic intervention [65,67].

measurements be interpreted using the total hip ROI and the hip BMD reference ranges derived from the third US National Health and Nutrition Examination Survey (NHANES III) [61].

NHANES III studied a nationally representative sample of over 14,000 men and women, with approximately equal numbers of non-Hispanic white, non-Hispanic black, and Mexican Americans. Data were gathered using DXA scanners operated from trailers so that subjects from all regions of the USA could be included. The ICSBM report recommends use of the total hip ROI instead of the previously widely used femoral neck site because of its improved precision and the fact that the hip region is the most readily implemented by all manufacturers' systems.

Many centers have acted upon these recommendations, and they are increasingly being used for scan interpretation. It is important to note that these changes affect the percentage of patients who are diagnosed as having osteoporosis at the hip. Using the total hip ROI and the NHANES III reference range, fewer patients will be diagnosed as having osteoporosis than when using the femoral neck ROI and the manufacturer's reference range [62]. There is no definite right or wrong answer in this situation. It is important, however, to have a consistent approach and it is certainly highly desirable to have universally accepted DXA BMD criteria for the diagnosis of osteoporosis.

One advantage of presenting bone densitometry results as T-scores is that they avoid the confusion caused by the raw BMD figures, which differ for different manufacturers' equipment [63]. The ICSBM has addressed this issue by publishing equations that allow each manufacturer to express their BMD values on a consistent scale in standardized units (sBMD: units mg/cm^2) [60,64]. Their report also included figures for the NHANES III total hip reference data converted into sBMD values.

Clinical decision making

With the development of new treatments for preventing osteoporosis, and the wider availability of bone densitometry equipment, much debate has centered on the issue of the clinical indications for the diagnostic use of bone densitometry, and recommendations for the initiation of treatment based on the findings.

1. **Presence of strong risk factors**

   Estrogen deficiency

   > Premature menopause (age <45 years)

   > Prolonged secondary amenorrhea (>1 year)

   > Primary hypogonadism

   Corticosteroid therapy

   > Prednisolone >7.5 mg/day for ≥1 year

   Maternal family history of hip fracture

   Low body mass index (<19 kg/m²)

   Other disorders associated with osteoporosis

   > Anorexia nervosa

   > Malabsorption syndrome

   > Primary hyperparathyroidism

   > Posttransplantation

   > Chronic renal failure

   > Hyperthyroidism

   > Prolonged immobilization

   > Cushing's syndrome

2. **Radiographic evidence of osteopenia and/or vertebral deformity**

3. **Previous fragility fracture, especially of the hip, spine, or wrist**

4. **Loss of height, thoracic kyphosis (after radiographic confirmation of vertebral deformities)**

Table 5.4 Risk factors providing indications for the diagnostic use of bone densitometry. Table reproduced from [66].

In the USA, an influential report was published by the National Osteoporosis Foundation (NOF) [65]. In Europe, similar reports were issued by the European Foundation for Osteoporosis [3], and by the Royal College of Physicians (RCP) in the UK [66].

The NOF report included a sophisticated set of guidelines for therapeutic intervention [65]. Various nomograms were developed that incorporated age, BMD, and four other risk factors for osteoporosis (**Table 5.3**). An interesting aspect of the NOF approach is that the calculations for therapeutic intervention were based on the concept of a quality-adjusted life year, costed at $30,000. This is a relatively high value, and one that would not be considered appropriate for application in Europe. This implies that there may have to be different BMD criteria for therapeutic intervention in different countries throughout the world. It also follows from the NOF approach that there will be different thresholds for intervention depending on the cost of treatment.

While the NOF report is an extremely important document, with an extensive review of the relevant background information, it is nevertheless complex, and it

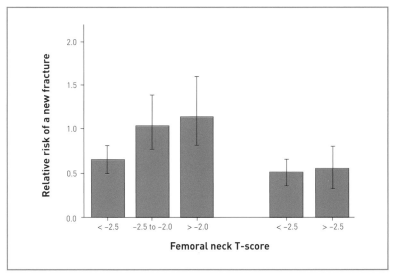

Figure 5.16 Results for fracture prevention from the Fracture Intervention Trial. The figure shows the ratio of the fracture incidence in the treatment and placebo arms of the study for: **(left)** any clinically presenting fracture (data from Cummings et al [45]); **(right)** vertebral fracture only (data from Black et al [76]). Results are shown plotted as a function of femoral neck bone mineral density T-score. For nonvertebral fractures, only patients who fulfill the World Health Organization definition of osteoporosis with a T-score of less than or equal to –2.5 show a statistically significant response to treatment.

is unlikely that primary care physicians will instigate treatment based on such a scheme. The NOF subsequently published a physicians' handbook with simplified recommendations that included the availability of BMD measurements for all women ≥65 years, and in all postmenopausal women <65 years in whom clinical risk factors are present [67]. The handbook recommends that treatment be considered for postmenopausal women with a T-score <–1.5 in the presence of one or more clinical risk factors for osteoporosis, and for women with a T-score <–2 regardless of risk factors.

In the UK, clinical guidelines for the prevention and treatment of osteoporosis have been published by the RCP [66,68]. These concluded that, at present, there is no consensus for a policy of population screening using BMD scans. Instead, a case-finding strategy is recommended for referring patients for bone densitometry based on a list of widely accepted clinical risk factors (**Table 5.4**). The RCP guidelines recommend a DXA T-score of less than or equal to –2.5 as the basis for instigating therapy.

It is important to emphasize that the WHO definition of osteopenia (–2.5<T<–1) is not useful in isolation with regard to decisions about treatment,

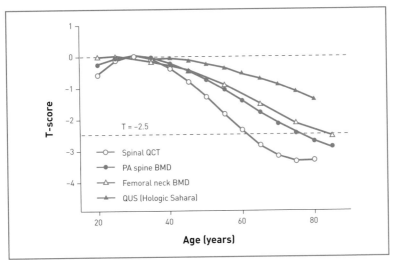

Figure 5.17 Age-related decline in mean T-score for white female subjects for: (1) spine dual-energy X-ray absorptiometry (DXA) – Hologic manufacturer's reference range; (2) femoral neck DXA (NHANES III reference range [61]); (3) spinal quantitative computed tomography (QCT) (data from Cann et al [77]); (4) quantitative ultrasound (QUS) of the calcaneus (data from Frost et al [78]). BMD: bone mineral density; PA: posteroanterior.

since it captures too high a percentage of postmenopausal women and was never intended to be used in this way. The evidence available from clinical trials indicates that patients with the most severe disease benefit most from treatment (**Figure 5.16**) [45,48]. In Europe, there seems to be a consensus supporting the use of a T-score ≤−2.5 as the appropriate intervention threshold for instigating treatment in white women.

However, it is important to take into account the other relevant clinical factors, such as those listed in **Tables 5.3** and **5.4**. In particular, the age of the patient and whether there is a history of previous fragility fractures are important independent predictors of future fracture risk. No consensus has yet emerged on which intervention thresholds are appropriate in men and other ethnic groups. However, the revised European guidelines published by Kanis and Glüer recommended that the same absolute BMD thresholds applied to white women should also apply to these other groups [69].

Views on how best to use BMD measurements when advising patients about the use of treatments to prevent fractures continue to evolve. Part of the limitation of T-scores is that the values obtained depend as much on the type of measurement as on the skeletal status of the patient, so the same threshold cannot be applied to all techniques (**Figure 5.17**). An alternative approach examined in recent analyses is to base treatment thresholds on estimates of

10-year fracture risk derived on the basis of age, BMD, previous history of fracture, and other clinical risk factors [40,41,70]. It seems likely that at some point in the future new guidelines will emerge, which will base treatment decisions on absolute fracture risk.

Follow-up DXA scans

Accuracy and precision

An important factor in the use of DXA scans for longitudinal studies is their relatively good precision. Like any physical measurement, BMD studies are affected by both accuracy and precision errors [71]. The accuracy of a technique reflects the degree to which the results deviate from the true values, while the precision reflects the reproducibility. Moderate accuracy errors in BMD scans, eg, those due to variations in soft tissue composition discussed above (typically 3–6%), may be acceptable, provided that they do not adversely affect the ability to diagnose osteoporosis. In contrast, for longitudinal studies it is the precision errors that are more important, since they represent a limitation on the smallest BMD change that can be regarded as statistically significant in follow-up studies.

The evaluation of precision

Precision errors are evaluated by performing repeated scans on a representative set of individuals, to characterize the reproducibility of the technique [71]. Most published studies examine the short-term precision error based on repeated measurements of each subject, performed over a time period of no more than 2 weeks. Over such a short period, no true change in BMD is expected. Precision results are expressed as the coefficient of variation (CV) by writing the SD as a percentage of the mean. Precision studies are usually performed by obtaining duplicate scans in a number of individuals, and data for at least 30 subjects are required to ensure reasonable statistical accuracy in the results [71]. The evaluation of long-term precision is complicated by the need to allow for the real changes in BMD that can occur over time periods of several years [72].

Longitudinal DXA scans in research studies

The past decade has seen the publication of data from many clinical trials and other research studies examining new pharmaceutical approaches to the prevention of osteoporotic fractures. Many recent trials using DXA have involved studies to evaluate bisphosphonates, such as alendronate [7,43–45] and risedronate [9,46,48], and data on the long-term effects of treatment are now available [44]. Other types of treatment for which large clinical trials have been published include calcitonin [47], the selective estrogen receptor modulator raloxifene [8], and parathyroid hormone [10].

Studies have also been conducted to establish the optimum dosage [8–10]. Research studies usually involve BMD scans of the spine and hip, since both are sites of clinically important fractures, and the spine is known to be the site that shows the largest response to treatment [21]. However, some studies have examined total body and forearm BMD as well. The number of subjects included in these studies is sufficiently large (often at least 100) to ensure that BMD changes as small as 1–2% are highly statistically significant.

Longitudinal DXA scans in individual patients
In many osteoporosis clinics, patients taking preventive treatment will have one or more follow-up scans, often at intervals of 1–2 years. Verifying response to treatment is widely believed to have a beneficial role in encouraging patients to continue taking their medication, and in ensuring that they are not continuing to lose bone.

The evaluation of changes seen on follow-up scans requires a knowledge of the smallest change in BMD that can be regarded as statistically significant, so that random measurement errors are not mistaken for real gains in bone mass [21]. The smallest significant change in BMD can be derived from the precision error of the technique expressed in terms of the CV. Because the initial baseline scan and the follow-up scan are both affected by these errors, the 1 SD difference between the first and second measurements will be $\sqrt{2}$ CV. The smallest change in BMD that is statistically significant with 95% confidence is therefore:

$$2 \times \sqrt{2} \times CV = 2.8 \times CV$$

Using long-term precision data, the figures for the smallest significant change are 4.6%, 6.9%, and 4.4% for spine, femoral neck, and total hip BMD, respectively [72]. These values can be compared with the results for the mean change in BMD with time reported by Tonino et al. for osteoporotic postmenopausal women treated with 10 mg alendronate daily over a period of 7 years [44]. On average, the 4.6% change required in spine BMD was reached 6–12 months after treatment was started, while the mean change in femoral neck BMD did not approach the required threshold level of 6.9%, even after 7 years of treatment. For some treatments, such as parathyroid hormone and the more potent bisphosphonates, statistically significant changes in spine BMD occur on time scales of 1–2 years in the majority of patients, while for other treatments the changes are often not large enough to be statistically significant.

Which measurement site is best for follow-up scans?
From the previous discussion of the smallest statistically significant change in BMD, it is clear that the choice of the optimum site for performing follow-up scans depends on the ratio of the BMD treatment effect to the precision of the measurements. The larger this ratio, the more statistically significant the observed changes will be. It follows that the ratio of treatment effect over precision is a useful index for comparing the merits of different measurement sites in the skeleton. **Figure 5.18** shows data for alendronate obtained from the Early Postmenopausal Intervention Cohort study [73,74]. The exact numeric results depend on the type of treatment, dosage, and the study population. However, all data agree in showing that the spine is the optimum site [21,73,75].

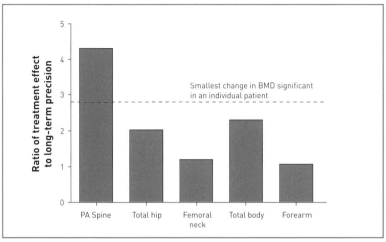

Figure 5.18 Ratio of mean change (difference between treated and placebo groups) in bone mineral density (BMD), divided by long-term precision for early postmenopausal women treated for 2 years with 5 mg/day alendronate or placebo at different skeletal sites. A statistically significant change of BMD in an individual patient requires a ratio of at least 2.8 ($p<0.05$). All studies to date agree in showing that the spine is the optimum site for follow-up BMD measurements. PA: posteroanterior. Data from the Early Postmenopausal Intervention Cohort study [73].

Conclusion

The 1990s saw increasing awareness of the clinical importance of osteoporosis and the validation of new treatments for fracture prevention (including the bisphosphonates, selective estrogen receptor modulators, and parathyroid hormone) in large-scale clinical trials. Alongside these developments, the pace of technologic innovation was rapid, with the introduction of new radiologic methods for the noninvasive assessment of patients' skeletal status. DXA scanning of the hip and spine remains the gold standard, although there is now a wider appreciation of the need for smaller, cheaper devices for scanning the peripheral skeleton if the many millions of women most at risk of a fragility fracture are to be identified and treated.

Several sets of guidelines for the clinical use of bone densitometry have been published, and most have included recommendations for intervention thresholds for initiating treatment in white women. Since the publication of the WHO report, opinion in Europe has increasingly favored the initiation of treatment following a diagnosis of osteoporosis based on a spine or hip T-score of –2.5 or lower. In the USA, the NOF suggests that treatment should be considered for postmenopausal women with a T-score $<$–1.5 in the presence of one or more clinical risk factors for osteoporosis, and for women with a T-score $<$–2, regardless of risk factors. However, care is needed in applying these figures to techniques other than DXA measurements of the spine, hip, or forearm, or in men or patients from other ethnic groups.

A concerted effort is being made to establish equivalent thresholds for other types of measurement, based on using femoral neck BMD as a gold standard. It is likely that, in the future, guidelines will be more orientated towards basing treatment decisions on estimates of absolute fracture risk using BMD and other risk factors, and that this approach will avoid some of the limitations of T-scores.

References

1. Genant HK, Engelke K, Fuerst T, et al. Noninvasive assessment of bone mineral and structure: state of the art. *J Bone Miner Res* 1996;11:707–30.
2. Baran DT, Faulkner KG, Genant HK, et al. Diagnosis and management of osteoporosis: guidelines for the utilization of bone densitometry. *Calcif Tissue Int* 1997;61:433–40.
3. Kanis JA, Delmas P, Burckhardt P, et al. Guidelines for diagnosis and treatment of osteoporosis. The European Foundation for Osteoporosis and Bone Disease. *Osteoporos Int* 1997;7:390–406.
4. Cooper C, Campion G, Melton LJ III. Hip fractures in the elderly; a world-wide projection. *Osteoporos Int* 1992;2:285–9.
5. Schurch MA, Rizzoli R, Mermillod B, et al. A prospective study on socioeconomic aspects of fracture of the proximal femur. *J Bone Miner Res* 1996;11:1935–42.
6. Ray NF, Chan JK, Thamer M, et al. Medical expenditures for the treatment of osteoporotic fractures in the United States in 1995: report from the National Osteoporosis Foundation. *J Bone Miner Res* 1997;12:24–35
7. Black DM, Cummings SR, Karpf DB, et al. Randomised trial of the effect of alendronate on risk of fracture in women with existing vertebral fractures. Fracture Intervention Trial Research Group. *Lancet* 1996;348:1535–41.
8. Ettinger B, Black DM, Mitlak BH, et al. Reduction of vertebral fracture risk in postmenopausal women with osteoporosis treated with raloxifene: results from a 3-year randomized clinical trial. Multiple Outcomes of Raloxifene Evaluation (MORE) Investigators. *JAMA* 1999;282:637–45.
9. Harris ST, Watts NB, Genant HK, et al. Effects of risedronate treatment on vertebral and nonvertebral fractures in women with postmenopausal osteoporosis: a randomised controlled trial. Vertebral Efficacy with Risedronate Therapy (VERT) Study Group. *JAMA* 1999;282:1344–52.
10. Neer RM, Arnaud CD, Zanchetta JR, et al. Effect of parathyroid hormone (1-34) on fractures and bone mineral density in postmenopausal women with osteoporosis. *N Engl J Med* 2001;344:1434–41.
11. Consensus Development Conference. Diagnosis, prophylaxis and treatment of osteoporosis. *Am J Med* 1993;94:646–50.
12. WHO Technical Report Series 843. *Assessment of fracture risk and its application to screening for postmenopausal osteoporosis*. Geneva: World Health Organization, 1994.
13. Heaney RP, Abrams S, Dawson-Hughes B, et al. Peak bone mass. *Osteoporos Int* 2000;**11**:985–1009.
14. Faulkner KG, von Stetton E, Miller P. Discordance in patient classification using T-scores. *J Clin Densitom* 1999;2:343–50.
15. Marshall D, Johnell O, Wedel H. Meta-analysis of how well measures of bone mineral density predict occurrence of osteoporotic fractures. *BMJ* 1996;312:1254–9.
16. Guglielmi G, Lang TF. Quantitative computed tomography. *Semin Musculoskelet Radiol* 2002;6:219–27.
17. Stewart A, Reid DM. Quantitative ultrasound in osteoporosis. *Semin Musculoskelet Radiol* 2002;6:229–32.18.
18. Mussolino ME, Looker AC, Madans JH, et al. Phalangeal bone density and hip fracture risk. *Arch Intern Med* 1997;157:433–8.
19. Jorgensen JT, Andersen PB, Rosholm A, et al. Digital X-ray radiogrammetry: a new appendicular bone densitometric method with high precision. *Clin Physiol* 2000;20:330–5.
20. Cummings SR, Black DM, Nevitt MC, et al. Bone density at various sites for prediction of hip fractures. The Study of Osteoporotic Fractures Research Group. *Lancet* 1993;341:72–5.
21. Eastell R. Treatment of postmenopausal osteoporosis. *N Engl J Med* 1998;338:736–46.
22. Njeh CF, Fuerst T, Hans D, et al. Radiation exposure in bone mineral assessment. *Appl Radiat Isot* 1999;50:215–36.
23. Blake GM, Herd RJ, Patel R, et al. The effect of weight change on total body dual-energy X-ray absorptiometry: results from a clinical trial. *Osteoporos Int* 2000;11:832–9.

24. Svendsen OL, Hassager C, Skodt V, et al. Impact of soft tissue on in-vivo accuracy of bone mineral measurements in the spine, hip, and forearm: a human cadaver study. *J Bone Miner Res* 1995;10:868–73.

25. Boudousq V, Kotzki PO, Dinten JM, et al. Total dose incurred by patients and staff from BMD measurement using a new 2D digital bone densitometer. *Osteoporos Int* 2003;14:263–9.

26. Melton L, Atkinson EJ, Cooper C, et al. Vertebral fractures predict subsequent fractures. *Osteoporos Int* 1999;10:214–21.

27. Genant HK, Jergas M, van Kuijk C. *Vertebral fracture in osteoporosis*. San Francisco, CA: University of California Osteoporosis Research Group, 1995.

28. Rea JA, Li J, Blake GM, et al. Visual assessment of vertebral deformity by X-ray absorptiometry: a highly predictive method to exclude vertebral deformity. *Osteoporos Int* 2000;11:660–8.

29. Rea JA, Chen MB, Li J, et al. Morphometric X-RAY absorptiometry and morphometric radiography of the spine: a comparison of prevalent vertebral deformity identification. *J Bone Miner Res* 2000;15:564–74.

30. Cameron JR, Sorensen J. Measurement of bone mineral in vivo: an improved method. *Science* 1963;142:230–2.

31. Düppe H, Gärdsell P, Nilsson B, et al. A single bone density measurement can predict fractures over 25 years. *Calcif Tissue Int* 1997;60:171–4.

32. Patel R, Blake G, Fogelman I. Radiation dose to the patient and operator from a peripheral dual X-ray absorptiometry system. *J Clin Densitom* 1999;2:397–401.

33. Bouxsein ML, Parker RA, Greenspan SL. Forearm bone mineral densitometry cannot be used to monitor response to alendronate therapy in postmenopausal women. *Osteoporos Int* 1999;10:505–9.

34. Kalender WA. Effective dose values in bone mineral measurements by photon absorptiometry and computed tomography. *Osteoporos Int* 1992;2:82–7.

35. Grampp S, Genant HK, Mathur A, et al. Comparisons of non-invasive bone mineral measurements in assessing age-related loss, fracture discrimination and diagnostic classification. *J Bone Miner Res* 1997;12:697–711.

36. Njeh CF, Hans D, Fuerst T, et al. *Quantitative Ultrasound: Assessment of Osteoporosis and Bone status.* London: Martin Dunitz, 1999.

37. Hans D, Dargent-Molina P, Schott AM, et al. Ultrasonographic heel measurements to predict hip fracture in elderly women: the EPIDOS prospective study. *Lancet* 1996;348:511–14.

38. Bauer DC, Glüer CC, Cauley JA, et al. Broadband ultrasonic attenuation predicts fractures strongly and independently of densitometry in older women. a prospective study. Study of Osteoporotic Fractures Research Group. *Arch Intern Med* 1997;157:629–34.

39. Pluijm SM, Graafmans WC, Bouter LM, et al. Ultrasound measurements for the prediction of osteoporotic fractures in elderly people. *Osteoporos Int* 1999;9:550–6.

40. Black DM. Revision of T-score BMD diagnostic thresholds. *Osteoporos Int* 2000;11(Suppl 2):S58 (abstract).

41. Blake GM, Knapp KM, Fogelman I. Absolute fracture risk varies with bone densitometry technique used: a theoretical and in-vivo study of fracture cases. *J Clin Densitom* 2002;5:109–16.

42. Black DM, Palermo L, Bauer D. How well does bone mass predict long-term risk of hip fracture? *Osteoporos Int* 2000;11(Suppl 2):S59 (abstract).

43. Liberman UA, Weiss SR, Bröll J, et al. Effect of oral alendronate on bone mineral density and the incidence of fractures in postmenopausal osteoporosis. The Alendronate Phase III Osteoporosis Treatment Study Group. *N Engl J Med* 1995;333:1437–43.

44. Tonino RP, Meunier PJ, Emkey R, et al. Skeletal benefits of alendronate: 7-year treatment of postmenopausal osteoporotic women. Phase III Osteoporosis Treatment Study Group. *J Clin Endocrinol Metab* 2000;85:3109–15.

45. Cummings SR, Black DM, Thompson DE, et al. Effect of alendronate on risk of fracture in women with low bone density but without vertebral fracture: results from the Fracture Intervention Trial. *JAMA* 1998;280:2077–82.

46. Reginster J, Minne HW, Sorensen OH, et al. Randomised trial of the effects of risedronate on vertebral fractures in women with established postmenopausal osteoporosis. Vertebral Efficacy with Risedronate Therapy (VERT) Study Group. *Osteoporos Int* 2000;11:83–91.

47. Chesnut CH III, Silverman S, Andriano K, et al. A randomized trial of nasal spray salmon calcitonin in postmenopausal women with established osteoporosis: the prevent recurrence of osteoporotic fractures study. Proof Study Group. *Am J Med* 2000;109:267–76.

48. McClung MR, Geusens P, Miller PD, et al. Effect of risedronate treatment on the risk of hip fracture in elderly women. Hip Intervention Program Study Group. *N Engl J Med* 2001;344:333–40.

49. Reid IR, Brown JP, Burckhardt P, et al. Intravenous zoledronic acid in postmenopausal women with low bone mineral density. *N Engl J Med* 2002;346:653–61.

50. Cummings SR, Palermo L, Browner W, et al. Monitoring osteoporosis therapy with bone densitometry: misleading changes and regression to the mean. *JAMA* 2000;283:1318–21.

51. Blake GM, Fogelman I. Peripheral or central densitometry: does it matter which technique we use? *J Clin Densitom* 2001;4:83–96.

52. Altman DG. *Practical Statistics for Medical Research*. London: Chapman & Hall, 1991.

53. Cummings SR, Black DM, Nevitt MC, et al. Appendicular bone density and age predict hip fracture in women. The Study of Osteoporotic Fractures Research Group. *JAMA* 1990;263:665–8.

54. Seeley DG, Browner WS, Nevitt MC, et al. Which fractures are associated with low appendicular bone mass in elderly women? *Ann Intern Med* 1991;115:837–42

55. Siris ES, Miller PD, Barrett-Connor E, et al. Identification and fracture outcomes of undiagnosed low bone mineral density in postmenopausal women: results from the National Osteoporosis Risk Assessment. *JAMA* 2001;286:2815–22.

56. Faulkner K, Abbott TA, Furman WD, et al. Fracture risk assessment in NORA is comparable across peripheral sites. *J Bone Miner Res* 2001;16(Suppl 1):S144 (abstract).

57. Massie A, Reid DM, Porter RW. Screening for osteoporosis: comparison between dual energy X-ray absorptiometry and broadband ultrasonic attenuation in 1000 perimenopausal women. *Osteoporos Int* 1993;3:107–10.

58. Rosenthall L, Tenenhouse A, Caminis J. A correlative study of ultrasound calcaneal and dual-energy X-ray absorptiometry bone measurements of the lumbar spine and femur in 1000 women. *Eur J Nucl Med* 1995;22:402–6.

59. Faulkner KG, Roberts LA, McClung MR. Discrepancies in normative data between Lunar and Hologic DXA systems. *Osteoporos Int* 1996;6:432–6.

60. Hanson J. Standardization of femur BMD [letter to the editor]. *J Bone Miner Res* 1997;12:1316–17.

61. Looker AC, Wahner HW, Dunn WL, et al. Updated data on proximal femur bone mineral levels of US adults. *Osteoporos Int* 1998;8:468–89.

62. Chen Z, Maricic M, Lund P, et al. How the new Hologic hip normal reference values affect the densitometric diagnosis of osteoporosis. *Osteoporos Int* 1998;8:423–7.

63. Genant HK, Grampp S, Glüer CC, et al. Universal standardization for dual X-ray absorptiometry: patient and phantom cross-calibration results. *J Bone Miner Res* 1994;9:1503–14.

64. Anon. Standardization of spine BMD measurements [letter to the editor]. *J Bone Miner Res* 1995;10:1602–3.

65. Anon. Osteoporosis: review of the evidence for prevention, diagnosis, and treatment and cost-effectiveness analysis. *Osteoporos Int* 1998;8(Suppl 4):S7–80.

66. Royal College of Physicians. *Osteoporosis: Clinical Guidelines for Prevention and Treatment*. London: Royal College of Physicians, 1999.

67. National Osteoporosis Foundation. *Physicians Guide to Prevention and Treatment of Osteoporosis*. Washington, DC: NOF, 1998.

68. Royal College of Physicians. *Osteoporosis: Clinical Guidelines for Prevention and Treatment. Update on pharmacological interventions and an algorithm for management*. London: Royal College of Physicians, 2000.

69. Kanis JA, Glüer CC. An update on the diagnosis and assessment of osteoporosis with densitometry. Committee of Scientific Advisors, International Osteoporosis Foundation. *Osteoporos Int* 2000;11:192–202.

70. Kanis JA, Johnell O, Oden A, et al. Ten year probabilities of osteoporotic fractures according to BMD and diagnostic thresholds. *Osteoporos Int* 2001;12:989–95.

71. Glüer CC, Blake G, Lu Y, et al. Accurate assessment of precision errors; how to measure the reproducibility of bone densitometry techniques. *Osteoporos Int* 1995;5:262–70.

72. Patel R, Blake GM, Rymer J, et al. Long-term precision of DXA scanning assessed over seven years in forty postmenopausal women. *Osteoporos Int* 2000;11:68–75.

73. Hosking D, Chilvers CE, Christiansen C, et al. Prevention of bone loss in postmenopausal women under 60 years of age. Early Postmenopausal Intervention Cohort Study Group. *N Engl J Med* 1998;338:485–92.

74. Faulkner KG. Bone densitometry: choosing the proper skeletal site to measure. *J Clin Densitom* 1998;1:279–86.

75. Blake GM, Herd RJ, Fogelman I. A longitudinal study of supine lateral DXA of the lumbar spine: a comparison with posteroanterior spine, hip and total body DXA. *Osteoporos Int* 1996;6:462–70.

76. Black D, Thompson D, Quandt S, et al. Alendronate reduces risk of vertebral fracture in women with BMD T-scores above –2.5: results from the Fracture Intervention Trial. *Osteoporos Int* 2002;13(Suppl 1):S27 (abstract).

77. Cann CE, Genant HK, Kolb FO, et al. Quantitative computed tomography for prediction of vertebral fracture risk. *Bone* 1985;6:1–7.

78. Frost ML, Blake GM, Fogelman I. Contact quantitative ultrasound: an evaluation of precision, fracture discrimination, age-related bone loss and applicability of the WHO criteria. *Osteoporos Int* 1999;10:441–9.

6

Biochemical Markers of Bone Turnover

Ramasamyiyer Swaminathan

Introduction

Bone is a metabolically active tissue that undergoes continuous remodeling, involving bone resorption and bone formation. These two processes are tightly coupled, which means that formation is linked to resorption through intricate mechanisms. The cells responsible for resorption and formation are osteoclasts and osteoblasts, respectively. Numerous factors, both systemic and local, regulate the function of these cell types. Bone remodeling takes place on the surface of bone and, in a typical remodeling cycle, resorption takes 7–10 days, while formation takes 2–3 months. Cancellous bone, which makes up 20% of bone mass, accounts for 80% of bone surface area and is therefore more metabolically active and undergoes more rapid remodeling. Every year, 25% of cancellous and 2–3% of compact bone undergoes remodeling. Bone consists of an organic matrix (the osteoid), minerals, and bone cells. Organic matrix comprises predominantly type I collagen (90%) with small amounts of other proteins, including osteocalcin (OC), osteonectin, and osteopectin.

Several techniques are available for studying bone. These include bone histomorphometry, densitometry, and measurement of biochemical markers. Biochemical markers reflect the processes involved in remodeling and are therefore useful in the management of metabolic bone diseases. Biochemical markers of bone turnover that can be measured in body fluids include:

- enzymes or proteins secreted by osteoblasts and osteoclasts
- breakdown products released during resorption
- by-products released during bone formation

These markers are usually classified as bone formation and resorption markers. Changes in bone remodeling are reflected early by resorption markers, as resorption is a shorter process than formation. Biochemical markers are noninvasive, and can reveal acute changes in bone turnover. In order to be useful, an ideal biochemical marker of bone turnover should: be specific for one of the metabolic processes in bone; have a known mode of clearance, metabolism, and plasma half-life; and be easily measurable and stable in serum or urine. No such ideal marker exists.

Markers of bone formation

Osteoblasts synthesize and secrete a number of proteins that can be measured in serum as markers of their activity, and therefore of bone formation. The most commonly used markers of bone formation are alkaline phosphatase (AP), OC, C-terminal propeptide of type I procollagen (PICP), and N-terminal propeptide of procollagen I (PINP). Bone sialoprotein (BSP) might also prove a useful marker (**Table 6.1**) [1,2].

Bone alkaline phosphatase

APs are plasma membrane enzymes. Four genes code for AP, giving rise to four isoenzymes:

- placental
- intestinal
- germ cell
- tissue nonspecific forms

Nonspecific AP is expressed in many tissues including the liver, bone, and kidneys. Most of the circulating AP is from bone and liver. The isoforms of AP from bone and liver differ in their carbohydrate attachment and the degree of sialation [3]. Bone AP has a half-life of 1–2 days. Total serum AP can be easily measured, but is of limited value in the management of osteoporosis. Until recently, the methods used for measuring bone AP were crude, often laborious, and imprecise. These methods were based on heat inactivation, chemical, or electrophoresis [3]. Precipitation of bone AP with wheat germ lectin provides a simple technique to quantitate bone AP. However, this method has poor reproducibility due to variation in different batches of wheat germ lectin.

Measurement of bone AP using antibodies specific for this isoform has now been developed. In these methods, mass of bone AP is measured by an immunoradiometric assay, or the activity is measured after capturing the bone AP using specific antibodies attached to a plate. These methods can be easily automated and have acceptable precision and reasonable specificity, although there is some cross-reactivity with the liver isoform [3]. Furthermore, as the bone isoform is cleared by the liver, it may be elevated in liver disease [1]. Bone AP measurements correlate with bone mineralization rates [4] and have been shown to respond to the treatment of osteoporotic subjects with alendronate [5].

Marker	Method	Sample	Specificity	Major source
Bone formation				
Total AP	CM	S	(+)	Liver/bone
Bone AP	CM/IA	S	++	Bone (osteoblasts)
Osteocalcin	IA	S/P	+++	Bone (osteoblasts)
PICP	IA	S	+	Bone (osteoblasts)
				Skin (fibroblasts)
Bone sialoprotein	IA	S	?	Bone (osteoblasts)
Osteonectin	IA	S	(?)	Bone (osteoblasts)
				Blood (platelets)
Bone resorption				
TRAP	CM/IA	S/P	++	Bone (osteoclasts)
Hydroxyproline	CM/HPLC	U	(+)	Connective tissue (collagen)
Hydroxylysine glycosides	HPLC	U	++	Connective tissue (collagen)
PYD	HPLC/IA	U	++	Bone and cartilage (collagen)
DPD	HPLC/IA	S/U	+++	Bone and dentine (collagen)
N-terminal telopeptide	IA	S/U	+++	Bone and dentine (collagen)
C-terminal telopeptide (cross-laps)	IA	S/U	+++	Bone and dentine (collagen)

Table 6.1 Summary of biochemical markers. AP: alkaline phosphatase; CM: colorimetric method; DPD: deoxypyridinoline; HPLC: high-performance liquid chromatography; IA: immunoassay; P: plasma; PICP: C-terminal propeptide of type I procollagen; PYD: pyridinoline; S: serum; TRAP: tartrate-resistant acid phosphatase; U: urine.

Osteocalcin

OC (or bone γ-carboxyglutamate [GLA] protein), a small, noncollagenous protein of molecular weight 5,800 kDa, is a unique product of osteoblasts and odontoblasts [2,4]. It is the most abundant noncollagenous protein in bone. The precise function of OC is unclear, although a possible role as a messenger in the coupling of osteoclast and osteoblast activities has been suggested [6]. It contains glutamic acid residues, which are converted to bone GLA protein by posttranslational vitamin K-dependent carboxylation. Most of the OC that is produced is incorporated into the bone matrix, where it is bound to hydroxyapatite; a small fragment is released into the circulation. The proportion of OC incorporated into the matrix varies from >90% in the young to 70% in

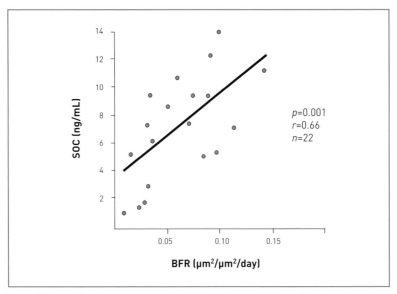

Figure 6.1 Correlation between serum osteocalcin (SOC) concentration and bone formation rate (BFR). Adapted from Delmas [9].

adults. The half-life of OC in the circulation is a few minutes, and it is rapidly cleared from the circulation by glomerular filtration.

Although OC and AP are the products of osteoblasts, concentrations do not always change in parallel, suggesting that they reflect different processes [7,8]. Serum OC concentration is a sensitive marker of bone formation and correlates with histomorphometric indices of bone formation (**Figure 6.1**) [9]. It is increased in conditions associated with increased bone turnover.

Although serum OC can be measured by readily available commercial immunoassay kits, comparison between methods is poor due to different antibodies recognizing different epitopes [10], instability of the molecule, and lack of an internationally agreed standard [10,11]. In serum, in addition to the intact molecule, several fragments are found (**Figure 6.2**) [10]. Analyses of the same samples by several commercial kits have shown a wide variation in results, although the methods were highly correlated (**Figure 6.3**) [10,12]. To avoid problems associated with OC fragments in the serum, most recently developed assays are two-site immunoassays designed to measure the intact protein. However, there is still considerable assay variability due to immunochemical heterogeneity.

Storage of samples can lead to cleavage of the protein, giving rise to a large N-terminal fragment (see **Figure 6.2**). Assays that measure intact OC and the

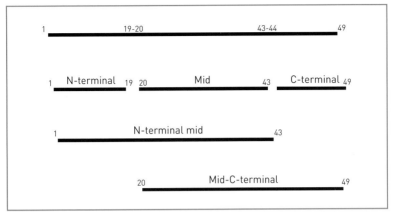

Figure 6.2 Heterogeneity of circulating osteocalcin. Reproduced with permission from the Royal Society of Medicine Services [10].

large N-terminal fragment are far less susceptible to changes during storage [13]. Blood samples for OC should be collected and packed on ice, have plasma or serum separated within an hour, and kept at –20°C for short-term storage and –70°C for long-term storage [10]. Samples should be thawed only once, to prevent degradation and generation of fragments. As OC is cleared by the kidneys, serum concentration can be increased in renal failure. However, it must be remembered that patients with chronic renal failure have increased bone turnover [2].

Procollagen I extension peptides

Type I collagen, which makes up 90% of the organic matrix of bone, is synthesized as a procollagen precursor molecule. The procollagen molecule contains extension peptides at both amino- and carboxy-terminal ends. These are cleaved by specific endoproteases before the collagen becomes incorporated into the bone matrix (**Figure 6.4**). These peptides (PICP and PINP) can be measured as markers of bone formation.

PICP

The trimeric PICP, which is stabilized by interchain disulfide bonds, has a molecular weight of approximately 100 kDa, is not filtered at the glomerulus, and is therefore not affected by renal function. The half-life of PICP is in the region of 6–8 minutes, and it is thought to be cleared through a specific receptor via the mannose-receptor pathway of the hepatic endothelial cell [14]. The ratio of collagen deposited in the bone matrix to PICP released into the bloodstream should be 1:1. PICP is stable in serum and it can be assayed confidently by immunoassay in specimens that have been frozen and thawed a number of times. It has also been shown that the molecule is stable at room temperature for up to 15 days. Serum concentrations of PICP correlate with other indices, such as bone

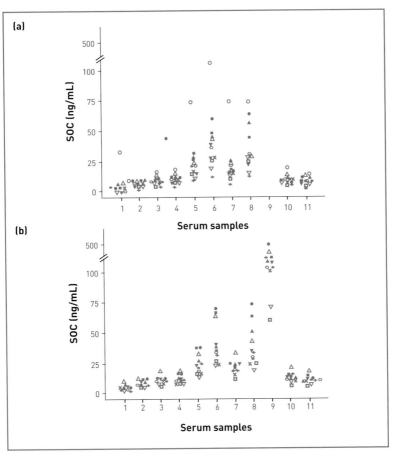

Figure 6.3 Concentration of serum osteocalcin (SOC) in 11 serum samples measured using different assays (represented by different symbols). **(a)** Results obtained using an in-house osteocalcin standard. **(b)** Results obtained with a reference standard. Reproduced from *J Bone Miner Res* 1990;5:5–11 with permission of the American Society for Bone and Mineral Research.

histomorphometry and whole body calcium kinetic indices [14,15]. However, this is not sensitive for detecting small changes in bone turnover, such as those seen during the menopause [16].

PINP

Immunoassays for the other extension peptide, PINP, have also been described. PINP circulates as two major components in serum, a 100 kDa and a 30 kDa component. The smaller molecule is thought to be a degradation product. Antibodies in different immunoassays react differently to these components, giving rise to differences in results between assays. Radioimmunoassay measures

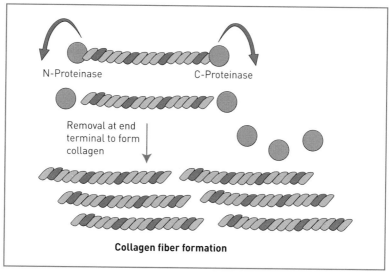

N-Proteinase   C-Proteinase

Removal at end
terminal to form
collagen

Collagen fiber formation

Figure 6.4 Procollagen extension peptides.

mainly the 100 kDa form of PINP [17]. An immunoassay that recognizes the intact molecule has been developed and has been found to be more sensitive than PICP for detecting changes in bone formation associated with the menopause and bisphosphonate treatment [18,19]. Several studies have shown PINP to be a useful marker of bone formation. For example, after surgical menopause, serum PINP was found to show the greatest change out of all the biochemical markers measured [20].

Bone sialoprotein
BSP, a glycosylated phosphoprotein of 80 kDa, is synthesized by osteoblasts and osteoclasts and accounts for 5–10% of noncollagenous protein of bone matrix. An immunoassay is available for its measurement, and serum concentration has been shown to be related to other established markers [21]. It has been shown to correlate better with bone resorption than formation [22]. Its usefulness in the management of osteoporosis has not yet been established.

Markers of bone resorption

Acid phosphatase
Acid phosphatases, a heterogeneous group of lysosomal enzymes, are present in many cells, including osteoclasts. The isoenzyme present in osteoclasts is resistant to tartrate (tartrate-resistant acid phosphatase [TRAP]). This enzyme, also known as type-5 acid phosphatase, is encoded by a gene located on chromosome 19 [2]. It is present in large quantities in the ruffled border of osteoclasts and is released during bone resorption.

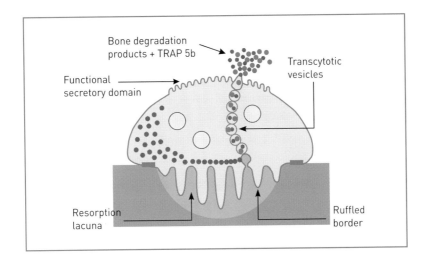

Figure 6.5 Release of tartrate-resistant acid phosphatase (TRAP) from osteoclasts.

During bone resorption, osteoclasts secrete acid and lysosomal proteins. The organic component of the bone is degraded by proteases and hydroxyapatite is dissolved by the acid. The matrix degradation products are endocytosed and fused with vesicles containing TRAP, which are then transported to the basolateral membrane where they are actively secreted through a functional secretory domain (**Figure 6.5**). TRAP further degrades the matrix components in the vesicles [23]. TRAP has also been identified in placenta and alveolar macrophages, and in the spleen of patients with Gaucher's disease and hairy cell leukemia. The isoform of TRAP present in osteoclasts has been identified as TRAP isoform 5b, which differs from the 5a isoform in its sialic acid content.

Serum TRAP can be measured by kinetic methods based on resistance to tartrate. However, the method has not been extensively studied as a marker of bone resorption, due to the fact that serum contains inhibitors of TRAP and due to interference from TRAPs derived from other cells such as erythrocytes and, possibly, platelets. The enzyme is also not stable in serum. The 5b isoform can be measured by a kinetic method [24].

Immunoassays based on antibodies raised against TRAP [25,26] or against the 5b isoform [27] have also been described. Using such assays, it was shown that the concentration of TRAP was higher in postmenopausal women and in situations associated with increased bone turnover [25,26,28]. Such immunoassays have also been found to be useful in predicting bone loss [29]. The full validity of these assays and their value in the management of osteoporosis needs to be further evaluated.

Hydroxyproline

Hydroxyproline (OHP), which represents about 13–14% of the amino acid content of collagen, is formed by posttranslational hydroxylation within the peptide chain. When collagen breaks down, OHP cannot be reutilized, and thus most of the OHP present in urine or serum is derived from collagen breakdown. As approximately half the total body collagen is present in bone, OHP excretion has been used as an index of bone resorption. However, urinary OHP is poorly correlated with the bone resorption rate and has now been largely replaced by more specific and sensitive assays [1,2].

Hydroxylysine

Hydroxylysine is another amino acid that is present in collagen, and, like OHP, is not reutilized in collagen synthesis. Hydroxylysine is present as galactosyl-hydroxylysine (GHYL) and glucosyl-galactosyl-hydroxylysine (GGHYL): the former is specific for collagen, while the latter is also present in molecules that have a collagen-like structure. Type I collagen in bone and skin differs in the structure of hydroxylysine glycosylation. GHYL predominates in bone, where the GHYL/GGHYL ratio is 7:1, while in the skin the ratio is approximately 1.6 [30].

The amount of hydroxylysine in collagen is much less than that of OHP, and the hydroxylysine concentration in urine is therefore much lower. However, neither GHYL nor GGHYL is present in procollagen peptides, and GHYL is therefore not released during bone formation. Furthermore, diet has no influence on the urinary excretion of these residues. These residues are not metabolized in the body and are excreted unchanged in the urine. As bone has higher concentrations of GHYL, it has been suggested that the excretion of GHYL might be a more specific index of bone resorption than OHP [30,31].

GHYL can be measured in the urine by high-performance liquid chromatography using a fluorometric detector, by an immunoassay [32], or by liquid chromatography/mass spectrometry [33]. The value of GHYL as a marker of bone resorption has not been fully evaluated. One study, however, found it to be a less reliable resorption marker due to its high biologic variation [34].

Collagen crosslink molecules

Type I collagen has a triple helix structure. The strands are connected by crosslinks between lysine or hydroxylysine residues that join the nonhelical end of one collagen molecule to the helical portion of the adjacent collagen molecule. There are two major crosslink molecules, pyridinoline (PYD) and deoxypyridinoline (DPD) (**Figure 6.6**) [35]. These are produced by posttranslational modification of lysine and hydroxylysine. These residues are the most important means of stabilizing collagen molecules by intramolecular crosslinks. Crosslinks are formed extracellularly after the deposition of collagen molecules into the matrix, and are released from bone only during bone resorption or collagen breakdown. PYD is widely distributed in connective tissue, including bone and cartilage (see **Table 6.1**) [1], the highest concentration

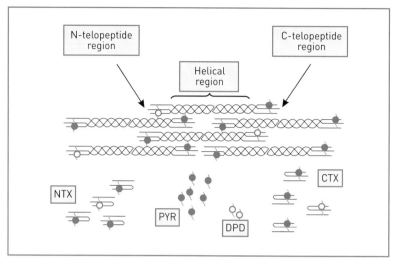

Figure 6.6 Type I collagen and crosslink degradation products. CTX: C-terminal telopeptide; DPD: deoxypyridinoline; NTX: N-terminal telopeptide; PYR: pyridinoline. Reproduced with permission from the American Association for Clinical Chemistry [1].

being in cartilage, whereas DPD is present in bone, dentine, the aorta, and ligaments. DPD constitutes approximately 21% of the total crosslinks in bone collagen [4].

DPD and PYD are released from bone in a ratio of 3:1. It is thought that PYD and DPD are not catabolized in the liver, but some of the pyridinoline crosslinks may be cleared through the liver. About 40–50% of the crosslinks are present in the free form, and 30–40% occur as very small peptide fragments (<1,000 MWt) and the rest as peptide fragments (1–10 kDa) [35]. The proportion of the free form in the urine is about 2-fold higher than in serum, suggesting that peptide-bound crosslinks are cleared in the kidneys to the free form [30]. As crosslink molecules are only found in mature collagen, the excretion of these molecules in the urine reflects the degradation of mature collagen and does not represent newly formed bone collagen [1].

PYD and DPD can be measured by high-performance liquid chromatography using a fluorescent detector, either after hydrolysis to measure the total or without hydrolysis to measure free crosslinks [36]. The free fraction can also be measured by enzyme immunoassay using monoclonal antibodies in serum or urine [35]. There is extensive literature suggesting that the excretion of crosslinks, especially DPD, is a good marker of bone resorption. The development of monoclonal antibodies [35] and a standard [37] will improve the usefulness of this assay, and the production of an immunoassay specific for the free form raises its wider accessibility. The excretion of collagen crosslinks in urine is

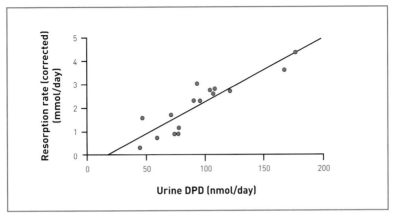

Figure 6.7 Relationship between bone resorptive rate and urinary deoxypyridinoline (DPD) in patients with osteoporosis. Data from Eastell et al [38].

increased in osteoporosis and in situations where bone resorption is increased, such as in hyperparathyroidism and hyperthyroidism. Urinary DPD is correlated to other indices of bone turnover measured by histomorphometry or calcium kinetics (**Figure 6.7**) [38].

Crosslinked telopeptides of collagen I

During bone resorption, only about 40% of the crosslinks are released as free pyridinium crosslinks. The remaining 60% are in the form of peptide-attached crosslinks [14]. Type I collagen has two crosslink-forming sites, one in the amino-terminal and the other in the carboxy-terminal region of the molecule (see **Figure 6.6**). Antibodies have been raised against both of the telopeptides, and immunoassays have been described to measure the N-terminal telopeptide (NTX), and the C-terminal telopeptide (CTX) (CrossLaps) in serum and urine [1,30,35]. Clinical studies of these assays appear to show them to be better than other markers at assessing bone resorption [1,35].

ICTP assay

Serum crosslinked carboxy-terminal telopeptide of type I collagen (ICTP) assay measures a component of the C-terminal telopeptide. This assay is convenient and appears to be sensitive for detecting changes in bone resorption due to pathological diseases such as bone metastases. Its use in osteoporosis has been disappointing.

NTX assay

The NTX assay, which is based on an antibody raised against a peptide isolated from the urine of a patient with Paget's disease, appears to measure all type I collagen degradation products. The assay reacts with several pyridinium crosslink-containing peptides. However, it does not recognize the crosslink itself.

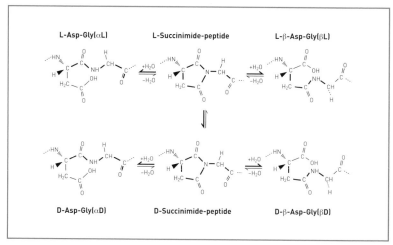

Figure 6.8 Structures of the isomerized and racemized -Asp-Gly- formed through succinimide intermediates in the telopeptide regions of type I collagen. Reproduced with permission from Elsevier [39].

This assay is unlikely to detect the degradation of newly formed type I collagen, since it does not react with the linear sequence of the telopeptide [30].

CTX assay

The assay for CTX was developed using antibodies against a synthetic peptide corresponding to the crosslinking site, and CTX can be measured in serum and urine [30]. It has been shown that proteins undergo posttranslational modification, and these are dependent on the age of the molecule. One such modification in type I collagen is the isomerization and racemization of aspartyl residues within the telopeptide region [39,40]. Detection of these isomers is of potential value. Immunoassays have been described to detect the native isoform (α-L) of CTX, and three age-related isoforms in urine. These age-related isoforms are β-L, α-D, and β-D, where the β denotes the isomerized structure, and D the racemized forms (**Figure 6.8**). In recent clinical studies, the α and β forms of all four isoforms have been measured [41–43]. The ratio of α-CTX to β-CTX has been found to be raised 3-fold in Paget's disease [44,45]. In women who have had a surgical menopause, levels of β-CTX were higher than those of α-CTX (although both were increased) [20].

It has been suggested that measurement of these isoforms may give an indication of the quality of bone [39]. The ratio of α-CTX to β-CTX was higher in postmenopausal women compared with premenopausal women, showing that bone turnover is quantitatively different in the postmenopausal stage [42]. In a prospective study to assess the risk of osteoporotic fracture (the OFELY [Os des Femmes de Lyon] study), Garnero et al. measured levels of all four isoforms of

CTX in the urine and found that a high ratio of native (α) to age-related CTX was associated with an increased risk of fracture, suggesting that changes in urinary isomerization/racemization of type I collagen may be associated with increased skeletal fragility [41].

Other assays

A urine assay detecting a degradation product from the helical part of type I collagen has now been described [46]. This assay was found to be a sensitive indicator of antiresorption treatment in postmenopausal women. An automated assay for serum CTX that recognizes β-aspartyl components has also been evaluated [47,48]. This assay uses two monoclonal antibodies to make it specific for β-CTX. Serum β-CTX measured by this assay showed a greater decrease compared with urine DPD in postmenopausal women treated with estrogens. High serum β-CTX was also associated with increased fracture risk [47]. It is difficult to compare the results of this assay with other previously reported results, as the units and standardization are different [39].

Recent studies on the use of these bone resorption markers suggest that urine NTX and serum CTX may be more sensitive than DPD in detecting changes during treatment [49].

Factors affecting bone markers

Analytic variability

One of the difficulties in translating the results of clinical trials into clinical practice is the analytic variability [50]. The problem of analytic variability is illustrated by the wide range of results for the same samples by different OC assays (**Figure 6.3**). An interlaboratory comparison of biochemical markers showed that, for the same sample, the difference between laboratories could be as high as 7.3-fold for bone AP and 5.6-fold for urine NTX [11]. One of the factors contributing to this difference is the lack of standardization. Different specificity of the antibodies used by different manufacturers, and sometimes by the same manufacturer, further complicates the picture.

For some assays (eg, for DPD) there have been attempts by international organizations to develop a standard to improve the situation [37]. The first step towards standardizing these assays was to agree upon the nomenclature [51]. For urine-based assays, the results are usually corrected for creatinine excretion. A study by Seibel et al. found that this led to a higher variation between laboratories [11]. In order to produce comparable results between laboratories, there should be cooperation between manufacturers and international organizations (such as the International Federation of Clinical Chemistry) to agree on standardization of methods and to develop robust external quality assurance programs.

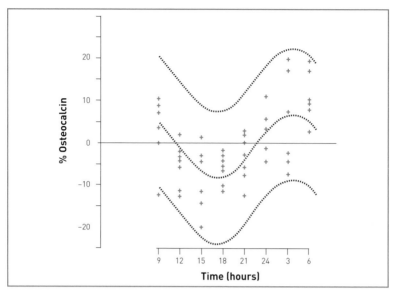

Figure 6.9 Diurnal variation in serum osteocalcin. Adapted from Eastell et al [95].

Preanalytic variation

Stability of samples

Another possible contributing factor to the variability of results is the stability of samples. Of the formation markers, OC is the most unstable at room temperature and at 4°C. It is also sensitive to freeze–thaw cycles [10]. Samples for OC should therefore be kept at 4°C after venepuncture, and serum or plasma should be separated as soon as possible and stored frozen [10].

Of the other markers, serum PINP and urine NTX were reported to be stable for 48 hours at room temperature and for 7 days at 2–8°C [52]. Urine DPD was not stable at room temperature, but was stable for 7 days at 4°C, and a recommendation to this effect has been published [53].

Intraindividual variation

Circadian cycle

Bone turnover shows a circadian rhythm, and this is reflected in biochemical markers [54]. Of the bone formation makers, OC shows a circadian rhythm, with a peak at 04.00 hours (**Figure 6.9**). Serum PINP and bone AP do not show this variation, probably reflecting slower clearance [55].

All bone resorption markers show a circadian pattern. DPD shows a variation of about 70% between the highest and lowest values [53]. Serum CTX shows the

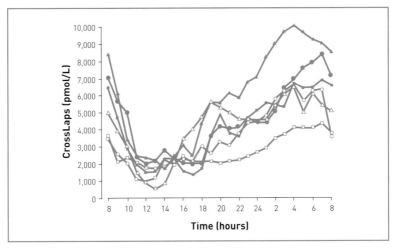

Figure 6.10 Diurnal variation of serum C-terminal telopeptide in six healthy male volunteers. Reproduced with permission from the American Association for Clinical Chemistry [56].

highest value at night between 01.30 and 04.30 hours, and lowest value between 11.00 and 15.00 hours, with about 120% difference between the highest and lowest values (**Figure 6.10**) [56]. The mechanism of this variation has been investigated and shown to be influenced by food intake [57], but not by bed rest, diurnal variation in cortisol, or by absence of a normal light cycle [58].

Day-to-day variability
All biochemical markers show marked day-to-day variation within the same individual. This variation is generally less for serum markers compared with urine markers [54]. The coefficient of variability is 5–13% for formation markers and 6–34% for resorption markers [59]. Feeding affects variability for some markers, especially serum CTX, and it has been suggested that, in order to minimize this, samples should be taken in the fasting state [60].

Physiological factors
Age, gender, and ethnicity may affect the results of measurement of bone markers. Bone AP and OC are lower in women than in men (<50 years). Serum OC was reported to be lower in black subjects compared with white and Mexican-American subjects, whereas bone AP was lower in white women compared with other groups [61]. Higher bone resorption markers in Arabic women have also been reported [62]. However, this difference between races could be due to variation in vitamin D status or other similar factors.

Critical differences
To use biochemical markers in practice, the magnitude of difference between two samples from a subject – which is not due to normal biologic and analytic

Marker	Critical difference (%)
Urine DPD	38
Urine NTX	40.6
Serum CTX	53.6
Serum PINP	38
Bone AP	24
Serum NTX	34

Table 6.2 Critical difference for some common biochemical markers of bone turnover. AP: alkaline phosphatase; CTX: C-terminal telopeptide. DPD: deoxypyridinoline; NTX: N-terminal telopeptide; PICP: C-terminal propeptide of type I procollagen; PINP: N-terminal propeptide of type I procollagen. Reproduced from Kyd et al [49] and Scariano et al [63].

variability – should be known. By determining the biologic and analytic variation, the coefficient of variation of critical difference can be calculated. The critical differences for some of the common markers are listed in **Table 6.2**.

In order to reduce the variation, samples should be collected at a specific time of the day – the most practical urine specimen is the second morning specimen [63].

Menopause

Bone turnover increases at menopause, as shown by histomorphometric and calcium kinetic studies [64]. As this is reflected in biochemical markers, serum concentrations of OC, PICP, CTX, and NTX, and urinary excretion of DPD, NTX, and CTX, all increase at menopause. However, the degree of elevation, even for the same marker, varies widely between studies. For example, serum OC has been reported to vary from 111% to 203% [2]. Some of this variation may be due to differences between assays (see section on analytic variation) or pre-analytic variation, and the rest may reflect the variation between individuals at menopause.

Of the markers of formation, bone AP measured by immunoradiometric assay has been found to show the greatest increase (204% compared with 150% for OC) [65]. Of the resorption markers, the greatest increases were seen in the newer markers: urine NTX (271%), serum CTX (254%), urine β-CTX (227%), and urine α-CTX (190%) [65–67].

Potential uses of bone markers in osteoporosis

Biochemical markers have only a minor role in the diagnosis of metabolic bone disease, especially osteoporosis.

Prediction of rate of bone loss

Theoretically, biochemical markers could reliably predict imbalance between bone formation and bone resorption, and therefore predict the rate of bone loss. If this is possible, it will provide a cheap and easy method to identify those at risk of developing osteoporosis. Several cross-sectional studies have shown a correlation between bone mineral density (BMD) at various sites and markers of bone turnover in postmenopausal women [30]. In older women, 30 years or more after the menopause, bone turnover accounts for 40–50% of the variation in BMD [68], suggesting that bone turnover rate could predict the rate of bone loss. In a cross-sectional study, PICP and OC were found to be better for predicting those with lower BMD [69,70]. In a similar study, Scariano et al. found that serum NTX and PINP had an overall diagnostic efficiency of 89% and 73%, respectively, in predicting low bone mass [71].

Longitudinal studies to show the predictive value of rate of bone loss from biochemical markers have shown conflicting results. Garnero and Delmas have commented that these studies are limited by the precision error of the measurement of BMD, which is of the same order of magnitude as the yearly rate of bone loss [30]. In a 12-year follow-up study, a combination of biochemical markers – AP, urinary calcium, and OHP – identified 'fast bone losers' [72]. In a later study, the same authors used OC, OHP, and DPD as markers, and showed a highly significant correlation between estimated and measured bone loss [73]. However, there have been very few long-term longitudinal studies to confirm this. In a study of 60 women over a 2–4 year period, Rogers et al. measured PINP, bone AP, OC, urine NTX, and free DPD, and showed that bone markers and rate of bone loss were correlated [74].

However, bone markers were not able to predict the rate of bone loss. In the Study of Osteoporotic Fractures, higher levels of urine NTX, CTX, DPD, and serum OC were associated with faster bone loss, but these were not specific or sensitive enough to predict bone loss [75]. In the Postmenopausal Estrogen/Progestin Interventions trial, NTX, and OC were related to BMD loss at the spine [76]. In the OFELY study, high urine and serum NTX and CTX were associated with rapid bone loss [77]. **Figure 6.11** shows the relationship between urine markers and change in BMD [75]. Although markers may predict bone loss in populations, they are less useful in the individual patient, due to the sources of variability previously mentioned.

Prediction of fracture risk

Patients with fractures show increased bone resorption and decreased bone formation [78]. However, these changes may be a response to the fracture. In an early study, high OHP at baseline was associated with a 2.8-fold increased risk of fracture in subsequent years [79]. More recent longitudinal studies have shown that baseline markers are predictors of subsequent fractures [80,81]. In the OFELY study, those with high markers of bone turnover were found to have an increased risk of fracture [81]. Measurement of bone density, together with bone

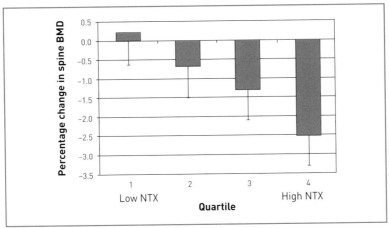

Figure 6.11 Relationship between baseline N-terminal telopeptide (NTX) and change in bone mineral density (BMD). Reproduced with permission from the American Association for Clinical Chemistry [1].

markers, improved the prediction value (**Figure 6.12**). In a 15-year follow-up study, those with increased bone turnover had a 2-fold higher risk of vertebral and peripheral fractures. If the higher bone turnover was associated with an initial low bone mass, the risk was even greater [82].

Urine CTX and DPD
In a French study of elderly women (Epidemiologie de l'Osteoporose [EPIDOS]), high baseline urine CTX and free DPD values were associated with a 2-fold increase in hip fractures. Although the sensitivity of high urine CTX to predict hip fracture was 36%, the specificity was 81%, and the positive predictive value was 3%. However, the combination of low BMD with high bone turnover has been shown to increase the predictive value [30].

OC and AP
In the Multiple Outcomes of Raloxifene Evaluation trial, a decrease in OC and bone AP after treatment with raloxifene was associated with a decreased risk of vertebral fracture [83]. **Figure 6.13** shows the probability of hip fracture when bone BMD and high CTX are combined in women of different ages [84].

OC is a vitamin K-dependent protein; in cases of vitamin K deficiency, it is not fully carboxylated. Under-carboxylated OC can be measured by a specific immunoassay. High serum under-carboxylated OC has been shown to be associated with an increased risk of subsequent fractures in elderly subjects [85,86]. Similar findings were reported in the EPIDOS study [87]. The risk of fracture was found to be higher if low BMD was associated with high under-carboxylated OC. High under-carboxylated OC might therefore reflect the

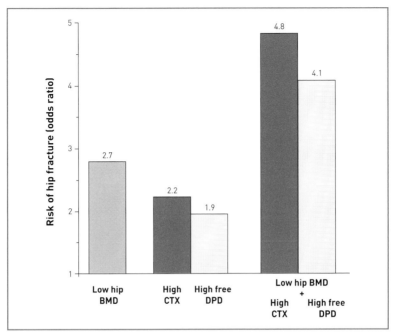

Figure 6.12 Risk of fracture at the hip according to low bone mineral density (BMD) and bone resorption rate. CTX: C-terminal telopeptide; DPD: deoxypyridinoline. Reproduced with permission from Elsevier [30].

quality of bone. In a study of children, under-carboxylated serum OC was correlated with ultrasound velocity, a measure of bone quality [88].

A study has reported that a high ratio of native (α-L) to age-related forms of CTX (β-L, α-D and β-D) indicated a 2-fold increased risk of fracture. The risk increased to nearly 5-fold if BMD was also low [45]. In spite of these promising results, markers cannot be recommended for routine use in clinical practice for predicting fractures.

Selection of treatment

In the treatment of osteoporosis, the aim is to reduce or prevent fractures. It has been suggested that the classification of subjects with rapid or slow bone turnover may help to determine the appropriate treatment – antiresorptive treatment for the former and anabolic agents for the latter. Until recently, this was only of theoretical interest, as most available treatments, such as bisphosphonates, calcitonin, and hormone replacement therapy, were antiresorptive. However, synthetic N-terminal fragment of parathyroid hormone (PTH1-34), an anabolic agent, has now been shown to increase BMD

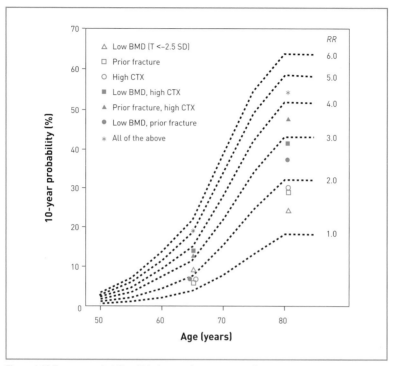

Figure 6.13 Ten-year probability of hip fracture in women according to age and risk factors.
BMD: bone mineral density; CTX: C-terminal telopeptide; RR: relative risk; SD: standard deviation.
Reproduced with permission from Springer Online [84].

substantially, and to be effective in reducing fracture rates [89]. This agent will soon be available for the treatment of severe osteoporosis. Biochemical markers could potentially be useful for identifying patients who may benefit from this treatment. However, as yet, there are no detailed prospective studies from which to make a judgement on this issue.

Predicting response to treatment

It has been suggested that baseline values for bone markers might predict the response to treatment [90]. Baseline NTX was found to correlate with change in BMD at 1 year (**Figure 6.14**). However, others have not been able to confirm these findings [1]. The large biologic variation in bone markers is one reason why bone markers may not accurately predict the response to treatment in an individual patient.

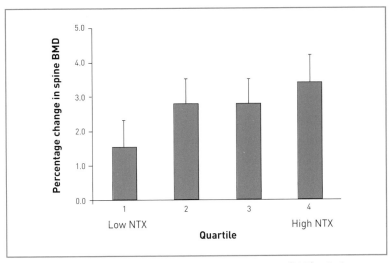

Figure 6.14 Relationship between change in spinal bone mineral density (BMD) and urine N-terminal telopeptide (NTX) in women receiving estrogen for 1 year. Reproduced with permission from the American Association for Clinical Chemistry [1].

Monitoring treatment

It is important to monitor the treatment of osteoporosis for two reasons.

- Firstly, to monitor compliance, which is not an uncommon problem, probably due to the side-effects of the drugs.
- Secondly, about 15–20% of patients do not respond to standard therapy [91].

Treatment can be monitored by repeating the measurement of BMD. However, due to the slow change in BMD (1–3% per year) and the precision of the available instruments, the interval between BMD measurements has to be ≥2 years.

Biochemical markers change more rapidly and may therefore be helpful in assessing the response to treatment. Several studies have found that changes in bone markers at 3 or 6 months correlate with changes in BMD at 2 years [19,92,93]. In a study of 120 elderly women treated with alendronate, changes in serum CTX and NTX at 6 months were correlated with changes in BMD at 2.5 years (**Figure 6.15**). However, the correlation coefficients were 0.42 and 0.31, respectively, and therefore are not adequate to predict changes in BMD. In a study of early postmenopausal women, changes in serum CTX were found to have a sensitivity of 49.5% in detecting improvement in bone density [92]. It has been suggested that the use of algorithms based on a spectrum of bone markers might be better for monitoring response [94].

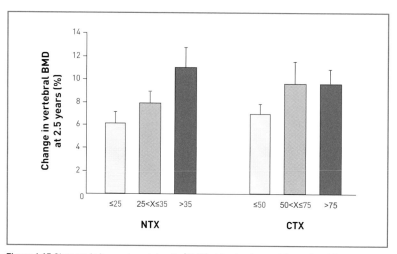

Figure 6.15 Changes in bone mineral density (BMD) at the lumbar vertebrae after 2.5 years of alendronate therapy according to percentage decrease in serum N-terminal telopeptide (NTX) and serum C-terminal telopeptide (CTX) at 6 months. Reproduced with permission from The Endocrine Society [92].

Advantages	Disadvantages
Noninvasive	Technical limitations
Easy to repeat	Storage stability
Large variation across the menopause	Variation between assays – precision, accuracy
Assess overall bone turnover	Lack of internationally agreed standards
Potential to study the pathogenesis	Diurnal variation
Potential to identify fast bone losers	Variation in metabolism and clearance
Early monitoring of therapy	Cannot localize the disturbance in bone metabolism

Table 6.3 Advantages and disadvantages of biochemical markers in studying bone turnover.

Conclusion

Biochemical markers have many advantages and disadvantages in studying bone turnover (**Table 6.3**). Many studies have shown that biochemical markers are useful in predicting bone loss and monitoring treatment. However, there is debate about the applicability of these markers in individual patients in clinical practice [50,91]. Factors contributing to this uncertainty are the large biologic variation in the markers and the lack of standardization of methodology [50], which gives rise to large interlaboratory variation.

Several new markers (such as the isomers of CTX) are currently under evaluation. Of the available markers, serum OC, bone AP, and PINP are useful markers of bone formation and DPD, NTX, and CTX are sensitive markers of bone resorption. Of the formation markers, bone AP or PINP are preferable, being more stable and showing less variation. Bone resorption markers can be measured in urine or serum. For both measurements, the timing of collection of samples has to be standardized, and in practice it may be more convenient to obtain a second void urine sample than to obtain a fasting sample at the clinic.

References

1. Watts NB. Clinical utility of biochemical markers of bone remodeling. *Clin Chem* 1999;45:1359–68.
2. Price CP, Thompson PW. The role of biochemical tests in the screening and monitoring of osteoporosis. *Ann Clin Biochem* 1995;32:244–60.
3. Price CP. Multiple forms of human serum alkaline phosphatase: detection and quantitation. *Ann Clin Biochem* 1993;30:355–72.
4. Calvo MS, Eyre DR, Gundberg CM. Molecular basis and clinical application of biological markers of bone turnover. *Endocrinol Rev* 1996;17:333–68.
5. Kress BC, Mizrahi IA, Armour KW, et al. Use of bone alkaline phosphatase to monitor alendronate therapy in individual postmenopausal osteoporotic women. *Clin Chem* 1999;45:1009–17.
6. Clowes JA, Eastell R. The role of bone turnover markers and risk factors in the assessment of osteoporosis and fracture risk. *Baillieres Best Pract Res Clin Endocrinol Metab* 2000;14:213–32.
7. Diaz-Diego EM, Diaz-Martin MA, de la Piedra C, et al. Lack of correlation between levels of osteocalcin and bone alkaline phosphatase in healthy controls and post-menopausal osteoporotic women. *Horm Metab Res* 1995;27:151–4.
8. Gundberg CM. Biochemical markers of bone formation. *Clin Lab Med* 2000;20:489–501.
9. Delmas PD. Biochemical markers of bone turnover in osteoporosis. In: Riggs BL, Melton LJ, eds. *Osteoporosis: Etiology, Diagnosis and Management.* New York, NY: Raven Press, 1988:297–316.
10. Lee AJ, Hodges S, Eastell R. Measurement of osteocalcin. *Ann Clin Biochem* 2000;37:432–46.
11. Seibel MJ, Lang M, Geilenkeuser WJ. Interlaboratory variation of biochemical markers of bone turnover. *Clin Chem* 2001;47:1443–50.
12. Masters PW, Jones RG, Purves DA, et al. Commercial assays for serum osteocalcium give clinically discordant results. *Clin Chem* 1994;40:358–63.
13. Blumsohn A, Hannon RA, Eastell R. Apparent instability of osteocalcin in serum as measured with different commercially available immunoassays. *Clin Chem* 1995;41:318–19.
14. Ristelli L, Ristelli J. Biochemical markers of bone metabolism. *Ann Med* 1993;25:385–93.
15. Charles P, Mosekilde L, Risteli L, et al. Assessment of bone remodeling using biochemical indicators of type 1 collagen synthesis and degradation: relation to calcium kinetics. *Bone Miner* 1994;24:81–94.
16. Hassager C, Fabbri-Mabelli G, Christiansen C. The effect of the menopause and hormone replacement therapy on serum carboxyterminal propeptide of type I collagen. *Osteoporos Int* 1993;3:50–2.
17. Brandt J, Krogh TN, Jensen CH, et al. Thermal instability of the trimeric structure of the N-terminal propeptide of human procollagen type I in relation to assay technology. *Clin Chem* 1999;45:47–53.
18. Garnero P, Vergnaud P, Delmas PD. Aminoterminal propeptide of type 1 collagen (PINP) is more sensitive marker of bone turnover than C-terminal propeptide in osteoporosis. *J Bone Min Res* 1997;12(SI):S497.
19. Fink E, Cromier C, Steinmetz P, et al. Differences in the capacity of several biochemical bone markers to assess high bone turnover in early menopause and response to alendronate therapy. *Osteoporos Int* 2000;11:295–303.
20. Peris P, Alvarez L, Monegal A, et al. Biochemical markers of bone turnover after surgical menopause and hormone replacement therapy. *Bone* 1999;25:349–53.
21. Fassbender WJ, Ruf T, Kaiser HE, et al. Serum levels of immunoreactive bone sialoprotein in osteoporosis: positive relations to established biochemical parameters of bone turnover. *In Vivo* 2000;14:619–24.
22. Seibel MJ, Woitge HW, Pecherstorfer M, et al. Serum immunoreactive bone sialoprotein as a new marker of bone turnover in metabolic and malignant bone disease. *J Clin Endocrinol Metab* 1996;81:3289–94.
23. Halleen JM, Raisanen S, Salo JJ, et al. Intracellular fragmentation of bone resorption products by reactive oxygen species generated by osteoclastic tartrate-resistant acid phosphatase. *J Biol Chem* 1999;274:22907–10.
24. Nakanishi M, Yoh K, Miura T, et al. Development of a kinetic assay for band 5b tartrate-resistant acid phosphatase activity in serum. *Clin Chem* 2000;46:469–73.

25. Cheung CK, Panesar NS, Haines C, et al. Immunoassay of a tartrate-resistant acid phosphatase in serum. *Clin Chem* 1995;41:679–86.

26. Alatalo SL, Halleen JM, Hentunen TA, et al. Rapid screening method for osteoclast differentiation *in vitro* that measures tartrate-resistant acid phosphatase 5b activity secreted into the culture medium. *Clin Chem* 2000;46:1751–4.

27. Miyazaki S, Igarashi M, Nagata A, et al. Development of immunoassays for type-5 tartrate-resistant acid phosphatase in human serum. *Clin Chem Acta* 2003;329:109–15.

28. Nakasato YR, Janckila AJ, Halleen JM, et al. Clinical significance of immunoassys for type 5 tartrate-resistant acid phosphatase. *Clin Chem* 1999;45:2150–7.

29. Rico H, Arribas I, Villa LF, et al. Can a determination of tartrate-resistant acid phosphatase predict postmenopausal loss of bone mass? *Eur J Clin Invest* 2002;32:274–8.

30. Garnero P, Delmas PD. Biochemical markers of bone turnover. *Endocrinol Metab Clin North Am* 1998;27:303–23.

31. Taylor AK, Lueken SA, Libanati C, et al. Biochemical markers of bone turnover for the clinical assessment of bone metabolism. *Rheum Dis Clin North Am* 1994;20:589–607.

32. Leigh SD, Ju HS, Lundgard R, et al. Development of an immunoassay for urinary galactosylhydroxylysine. *J Immunol Methods* 1998;220:169–78.

33. Casetta B, Romanello M, Moro L. A rapid and simple method for quantitation of urinary hydroxylysyl glycosides, indicators of collagen turnover, using liquid chromatography/tandem mass spectrometry. *Rapid Commun Mass Spectrom* 2000;14:2238–41.

34. Plebani M, Bernardi D, Meneghetti MF, et al. Biological variability in assessing the clinical value of biochemical markers of bone turnover. *Clin Chem Acta* 2000;299:77–86.

35. Robins SP. Biochemical markers of bone metabolism. *CPD Bulletin Clin Biochem* 1999;1:116–21.

36. James IT, Walne AJ, Perrett D. The measurement of pyridinium crosslinks: a methodological overview. *Ann Clin Biochem* 1996;33:397–420.

37. Robins SP, Duncan A, Wilson W, et al. Standardization of the pyridinium crosslinks, pyridinoline and deoxypyridinoline for use as biochemical markers of collagen degradation. *Clin Chem* 1996;42:1621–6.

38. Eastell R, Hampton L, Colwell A, et al. Urinary collagen crosslinks are highly correlated with radioisotopic measurements of bone resorption. In: Christiansen C, Overgaard K, eds. *Osteoporosis 1990*. Copenhagen: Osteopress, 1990: 469–77.

39. Robins SP. Collagen turnover in bone diseases. *Curr Opin Clin Nutr Metab Care* 2003;6:65–71.

40. Cloos PA, Fledelius C. Collagen fragments in urine derived from bone resorption are highly racemized and isomerized: a biological clock of protein aging with clinical potential. *Biochem J* 2000;345:473–80.

41. Garnero P, Cloos P, Sornay-Rendu E, et al. Type I collagen racemization and isomerization and the risk of fracture in postmenopausal women: the OFELY prospective study. *J Bone Miner Res* 2002;17:826–33.

42. Reginster JY, Henrotin Y, Christiansen C, et al. Bone resorption in post-menopausal women with normal and low BMD assessed with biochemical markers specific for telopeptide derived degradation products of collagen type I. *Calcif Tissue Int* 2001;69:130–7.

43. Cloos PA, Fledelius C, Christgau S, et al. Investigation of bone disease using isomerized and racemized fragments of type I collagen. *Calcif Tissue Int* 2003;72:8–17.

44. Vergnaud P, Lunt M, Scheidt-Nave C, et al. Is the predictive power of previous fractures for new spine and non-spine fractures associated with biochemical evidence of altered bone remodeling? The EPOS study. European Prospective Osteoporosis Study. *Clin Chem Acta* 2002;322:121–32.

45. Peris P, Alvarez L, Monegal A, et al. Effect of surgical menopause and Paget's disease of bone on the isomerization of type I collagen carboxyterminal telopeptide: evolution after antiresorptive therapy. *J Bone Miner Metab* 2002;20:116–20.

46. Garnero P, Delmas PD. An immunoassay for type I collagen alpha1 helicoidal peptide 620-633, a new marker of bone resorption in osteoporosis. *Bone* 2003;32:20–6.

47. Garnero P, Borel O, Delmas PD. Evaluation of a fully automated serum assay for C-terminal cross-linking telopeptide of type I collagen in osteoporosis. *Clin Chem* 2001;47:694–702.

48. Okabe R, Nakatsuka K, Inaba M, et al. Clinical evaluation of the Elecsys beta-CrossLaps serum assay, a new assay for degradation products of type I collagen C-telopeptides. *Clin Chem* 2001;47:1410–14.

49. Kyd PA, Vooght K, Kershoff F, et al. Clinical usefulness of biochemical resorption markers in osteoporosis. *Ann Clin Biochem* 1999;36:483–91.

50. Kleerekoper M. Biochemical markers of bone turnover: why theory, research, and clinical practice are still in conflict. *Clin Chem* 2001;47:1347–9.

51. Delmas PD. Standardization of bone marker nomenclature. *Clin Chem* 2001;47:1497.

52. Lomeo A, Bolner A. Stability of several biochemical markers of bone metabolism. *Clin Chem* 2000;46:1200–2.

53. Vesper HW, Demers LM, Eastell R, et al. Assessment and recommendations on factors contributing to preanalytic variability of urinary pyridinoline and deoxypyridinoline. *Clin Chem* 2002;48:220–35.

54. Hart SM, Eastell R. Biochemical markers of bone turnover. *Curr Opin Nephrol Hypertens* 1999;8:421–7.

55. Wolthers OD, Heuck C, Heickendorff L. Diurnal variations in serum and urine markers of type I and type III collagen turnover in children. *Clin Chem* 2001;47:1721–2.

56. Wichers M, Schmidt E, Bidlingmaier F, et al. Diurnal rhythm of cross laps in human serum. *Clin Chem* 1999;45:1858–60.

57. Bjarnason NH, Henriksen EE, Alexandersen P, et al. Mechanism of circadian variation in bone resorption. *Bone* 2002;30:307–13.

58. Qvist P, Christgau S, Pedersen BJ, et al. Circadian variation in the serum concentration of C-terminal telopeptide of type I collagen (serum CTx): effects of gender, age, menopausal status, posture, daylight, serum cortisol, and fasting. *Bone* 2002;31:57–61.

59. Hannon R, Eastell R. Preanalytic variability of biochemical markers of bone turnover. *Osteoporos Int* 2000;11(Suppl 6):S30–44.

60. Clowes JA, Hannon RA, Yap TS, et al. Effect of feeding on bone turnover markers and its impact on biological variability of measurements. *Bone* 2002;30:886–90.

61. Gundberg CM, Looker AC, Nieman SD, et al. Patterns of osteocalcin and bone specific alkaline phosphatase by age, gender, and race or ethnicity. *Bone* 2002;31:703–8.

62. Miller CJ, Dunn EV, Thomas EJ, et al. Urinary free deoxypyridinoline excretion in lactating and non-lactating Arabic women of the United Arab Emirates. *Ann Clin Biochem* 2003;40:394–7.

63. Scariano JK, Garry PJ, Montoya GD, et al. Critical differences in the serial measurement of three biochemical markers of bone turnover in the sera of pre- and postmenopausal women. *Clin Biochem* 2001;34:639–44.

64. Demers LM, Kleerekoper M. Recent advances in biochemical markers of bone turnover. *Clin Chem* 1994;40:1994–5.

65. Garnero P, Shih WJ, Gineyts E, et al. Comparison of new biochemical markers of bone turnover in late postmenopausal osteoporotic women in response to alendronate treatment. *J Clin Endocrinol Metab* 1994;79:1693–700.

66. Garnero P, Gineyts E, Riou JP, et al. Assessment of bone resorption with a new marker of collagen degradation in patients with metabolic bone disease. *J Clin Endocrinol Metab* 1994;79:780–5.

67. Kawana K, Takahashi M, Hoshino H, et al. Comparison of serum and urinary C-terminal telopeptide of type I collagen in aging, menopause and osteoporosis. *Clin Chem Acta* 2002;316:109–15.

68. Garnero P, Sornay-Rendu E, Chapuy MC, et al. Increased bone turnover in late postmenopausal women is a major determinant of osteoporosis. *J Bone Miner Res* 1996;11:337–49.

69. Majkic-Singh N, Ilic M, Ignjatovic S, et al. Assessment of four biochemical markers of bone metabolism in postmenopausal osteoporosis. *Clin Lab* 2002;48:407–13.

70. De Leo V, Ditto A, La Marca A, et al. Bone mineral density and biochemical markers of bone turnover in peri- and postmenopausal women. *Calcif Tissue Int* 2000;66:263–7.

71. Scariano JK, Garry PJ, Montoya GD, et al. Diagnostic efficacy of serum cross-linked N-telopeptide (NTx) and aminoterminal procollagen extension propeptide (PINP) measurements for identifying elderly women with decreased bone mineral density. *Scand J Clin Lab Invest* 2002;62:237–43.

72. Hansen MA, Overgaard K, Riis BJ, et al. Role of peak bone mass and bone loss in postmenopausal osteoporosis: 12 year study. *BMJ* 1991;303:961–4.

73. Delmas PD. What do we know about biochemical bone markers? *Baillieres Clin Obstet Gynaecol* 1991;5:817–30.

74. Rogers A, Hannon RA, Eastell R. Biochemical markers as predictors of rates of bone loss after menopause. *J Bone Miner Res* 2000;15:1398–404.

75. Bauer DC, Sklarin PM, Stone KL, et al. Biochemical markers of bone turnover and prediction of hip bone loss in older women: the Study of Osteoporotic Fractures. *J Bone Miner Res* 1999;14:1404–10.

76. Marcus R, Holloway L, Wells B, et al. The relationship of biochemical markers of bone turnover to bone density changes in postmenopausal women: results from the Postmenopausal Estrogen/Progestin Interventions (PEPI) trial. *J Bone Miner Res* 1999;14:1583–95.

77. Garnero P, Sornay-Rendu E, DuBoeuf F, et al. Markers of bone turnover predict postmenopausal forearm bone loss over 4 years: the OFELY study. *J Bone Miner Res* 1999;14:1614–21.

78. Cheung CK, Panesar NS, Lau E et al. Increased bone resorption and decreased bone formation in Chinese patients with hip fracture. *Calcif Tissue Int* 1995;56:374–9.

79. Woo J, Lau E, Swaminathan R et al. Biochemical predictors for osteoporotic fractures in elderly Chinese – a longitudinal study. *Gerontology* 1990;36:55–8.

80. Garnero P, Sornay-Rendu E, Claustrat B, et al. Biochemical markers of bone turnover, endogenous hormones and the risk of fracture in postmenopausal women: the OFELY study. *J Bone Miner Res* 2000;15:1526–36.

81. Tromp AM, Ooms ME, Popp-Snijders C, et al. Predictors of fractures in elderly women. *Osteoporos Int* 2000;11:134–40.

82. Riis BJ, Hansen MA, Jensen AM, et al. Low bone mass and fast rate of bone loss at menopause: equal risk factors for future fracture: a 15-year follow-up study. *Bone* 1996;19:9–12.

83. Bjarnason NH, Sarkar S, Duong T, et al. Six and twelve month changes in bone turnover are related to reduction in vertebral fracture risk during 3 years of raloxifene treatment in postmenopausal osteoporosis. *Osteoporos Int* 2001;12:922–30.

84. Johnell O, Oden A, De Laet C, et al. Biochemical indices of bone turnover and the assessment of fracture probability. *Osteoporos Int* 2002;13:523–6.

85. Szulc P, Chapuy MC, Meunier PJ, et al. Serum undercarboxylated osteocalcin is a marker of the risk of hip fracture: a three year follow-up study. *Bone* 1996;18:487–8.

86. Luukinen H, Kakonen SM, Pettersson K, et al. Strong prediction of fractures among older adults by the ratio of carboxylated to total serum osteocalcin. *J Bone Miner Res* 2000;15:2473–8.

87. Vergnaud P, Garnero P, Meunier PJ, et al. Undercarboxylated osteocalcin measured with a specific immunoassay predicts hip fracture in elderly women: the EPIDOS Study. *J Clin Endocrinol Metab* 1997;82:719–24.

88. Sugiyama T, Kawai S. Carboxylation of osteocalcin may be related to bone quality: a possible mechanism of bone fracture prevention by vitamin K. *J Bone Miner Metab* 2001;19:146–9.

89. Watts NB. Efficacy of teriparatide and alendronate on nonvertebral fractures. *J Clin Endocrinol Metab* 2003;8:1402–3.

90. Chesnut CH III, Bell NH, Clark GS, et al. Hormone replacement therapy in postmenopausal women: urinary N-telopeptide of type I collagen monitors therapeutic effect and predicts response of bone mineral density. *Am J Med* 1997;102:29–37.

91. Riggs BL. Are biochemical markers for bone turnover clinically useful for monitoring therapy in individual osteoporotic patients? *Bone* 2000;26:551–2.

92. Greenspan SL, Rosen HN, Parker RA. Early changes in serum N-telopeptide and C-telopeptide cross-linked collagen type 1 predict long-term response to alendronate therapy in elderly women. *J Clin Endocrinol Metab* 2000;85:3537–40.

93. Bjamason NH, Christiansan C. Early response in biochemical markers predicts long-term response in bone mass during hormone replacement therapy in early postmenopausal women. *Bone* 2000;26:561–9.

94. Ebeling PR, Akesson K. Role of biochemical markers in the management of osteoporosis. *Best Pract Res Clin Rheumatol* 2001;15:385–400.

95. Eastell R, Simmons PS, Colwell A, et al. Nyctohemeral changes in bone turnover assessed by serum bone Gla-protein concentration and urinary deoxypyridinoline excretion: effects of growth and ageing. *Clin Sci (Lond)* 1992;83:375–82.

7

Treatment of Established Osteoporosis

Judith Bubbear, Ajay Bhatia, and Richard Keen

Introduction

Osteoporosis is a systemic skeletal disease characterized by low bone mineral density (BMD), microarchitectural deterioration of bone tissue, and an increase in fracture risk [1]. The clinical significance of osteoporosis lies in the fractures that arise. The common osteoporotic-related fractures occur at the wrist (Colles' fracture), spine, and hip, and it is currently estimated that over 250,000 fractures per annum in the UK are attributable to osteoporosis [2]. A 50-year-old woman has an average lifetime risk of 17.5% for sustaining a hip fracture and 16% for sustaining a distal forearm fracture [3].

The aim of management in this condition is therefore to reduce the risk of future fracture. Strategies for the prevention or treatment of osteoporosis include population-based strategies and strategies targeted to people at high risk. There is limited evidence for a population-based approach having a significant impact on fracture risk, and published guidelines on disease management do not recommend this approach [4].

Treatment strategies for this condition have also evolved, based on both an improved understanding of the disordered pathophysiologic processes and on advances in pharmaceutical agents. The properties of ideal therapeutic agents are listed in **Table 7.1**.

Well tolerated	Safe
Increase bone mass	Restore normal bone architecture
Improve bone quality	Reduce fractures at all sites
Oral bioavailability	

Table 7.1 Properties of ideal therapeutic agents for osteoporosis.

Grade	Study design
Grade A	
Ia	Meta-analysis of RCTs
Ib	At least one RCT
Grade B	
IIa	Well designed, controlled trial
IIb	Well designed, quasi-experimental design
III	Case-control, comparative, or correlation studies
Grade C	
IV	Expert opinion/reports

Table 7.2 Levels of evidence. RCT: randomized controlled trial.

Agent		Fracture site	
	Vertebral	Nonvertebral	Hip
Alendronate	A	A	A
Calcitonin	A	B	B
Calcitriol	A	A	nd
Calcium	A	B	B
Calcium + vitamin D	nd	A	A
Etidronate	A	B	B
Hip protectors	–	–	A
HRT	A	A	A
Ibandronate	A	A	nd
Pamidronate (oral)	A	nd	nd
PTH	A	A	nd
Physical exercise	nd	B	B
Raloxifene	A	nd	nd
Risedronate	A	A	A
Strontium	A	A	A
Tibolone	nd	nd	nd
Vitamin D	nd	B	B
Zoledronate	nd	nd	nd

Table 7.3 Evidence base for agents in the management of postmenopausal osteoporosis.
HRT: hormone replacement therapy; nd: not demonstrated; PTH: parathyroid hormone.

A growing number of agents are available for the management of osteoporosis. Most of these have been studied in postmenopausal osteoporosis, and only a limited number of drugs are licensed for the treatment of osteoporosis in men. The evidence for these agents in reducing the risk of fracture at both vertebral and nonvertebral sites is given in **Tables 7.2** and **7.3**.

Nonpharmacologic treatment

General lifestyle measures should be adopted in all subjects at risk for osteoporosis. Many of these interventions are based on epidemiologic data linking either deficiency or excess of a particular factor with an increased risk of fracture. It is less clear, however, whether modification of the epidemiologic factor will result in a reduced fracture risk.

Diet

An optimal diet for the management of osteoporosis includes an adequate intake of calories (to avoid malnutrition), calcium, and vitamin D. In general, adults with osteoporosis require a dietary calcium intake of 1,000–1,500 mg/day, and this can be achieved either through the diet or with a formal supplement. An adequate vitamin D intake is also necessary for optimal bone health. Excess alcohol consumption appears to have a negative effect on bone health, both directly and also indirectly by increasing the risk of falls.

Smoking

Cigarette smoking is associated with reduced bone mass and an increased risk of fracture [5]. Subjects who are concerned about their skeletal health should be strongly encouraged to stop smoking.

Exercise

Regular weight-bearing exercise is encouraged to improve BMD. Any fracture reduction associated with exercise is probably a result of improved muscle strength and a lower risk of falling, particularly in the elderly. Excessive exercise in premenopausal women may actually have detrimental effects on bone, due to weight loss and secondary amenorrhea.

There is no evidence from controlled trials to suggest that exercise programs reduce the risk of fracture. Exercise can, however, reduce the risk of falls by about 25% in frail, elderly individuals [6]. In addition to exercise, individuals should also undergo a fall assessment, where risk factors for falls are identified and, where possible, reduced. These programs are being developed following the publication in the UK of the National Service Framework for Older People, and aim to identify subjects who are at high risk for falling, with the aim of adopting measures that will reduce their risk for injury.

Hip protectors

Controlled studies conducted in care homes have demonstrated that a structured education program and the provision of hip protectors can reduce the number of hip fractures [7]. Compliance with hip protectors is often poor; reasons cited for not wearing hip protectors include the physical difficulty of putting them on, urinary incontinence, and that they are too uncomfortable [8]. Better design and newer materials may reduce the noncompliance rate and make hip protectors more acceptable.

Group		Daily calcium intake (mg)
Infants	Birth–6 months	400
	6 months–1 year	600
Children	1–5 years	800
	6–10 years	800–1,200
Adolescents/young adults	11–24 years	1,200–1,500
Men	25–65 years	1,000
	>65 years	1,500
Women	25–50 years	1,000
	>50 years (postmenopausal)	
	• on estrogens	1,000
	• not on estrogens	1,500
	Pregnant and nursing	1,500
	>65 years	1,200–1,500

Table 7.4 Optimal calcium requirements.

Orthopedic management

Early surgical management of hip fractures is essential to decrease the mortality rate and improve postoperative mortality. There are no specific issues related to the management of peripheral fractures, as fracture healing rates are similar between patients with osteoporosis and age-matched controls.

Painful vertebral fractures may require specific attention. Historical treatments consisted of wearing corsets or surgical spinal braces, but this practice has now become outdated, as early mobilization is encouraged after the acute event. Active physiotherapy is of benefit, and analgesia can be provided by simple analgesics, transcutaneous electrical nerve stimulation (TENS), acupuncture, injectable/intranasal calcitonin, and intravenous bisphosphonate therapy. More recently, it has been suggested that vertebroplasty can relieve pain associated with a vertebral fracture. This technique involves the injection of polymethylmethacrylate cement into the vertebral body [9]. In the UK, the National Institute for Clinical Excellence (NICE) has reviewed percutaneous vertebroplasty, and supports the use of this technique in patients with vertebral fracture whose pain is refractory to more conservative treatment [10]. However, further controlled studies of this technique are required to better evaluate its long-term efficacy and safety. Balloon kyphoplasty is another technique that aims to restore vertebral height and reduce pain following fracture. Preliminary studies support its use [11]. Further studies will be required and NICE currently does not recommend its use [12].

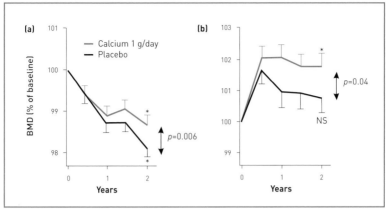

Figure 7.1 Effect of calcium (1 g) on postmenopausal bone loss. **(a)** Total body; **(b)** lumbar spine. The results are expressed as a percentage of the baseline values. Age of patients = 58+5 years. *$p<0.01$ versus baseline. BMD: bone mineral density; NS: not significant. Adapted from Reid et al [14].

Pharmacologic treatments

Calcium and vitamin D

Adequate calcium nutrition is essential for the development and maintenance of a normal skeleton (**Table 7.4**). At present, calcium supplements are often administered as a combined therapy with other agents for the treatment of osteoporosis. Vitamin D acts to increase calcium absorption in the gastrointestinal tract and thereby inhibits parathyroid hormone (PTH)-mediated bone resorption. The recommended daily requirement for calcium intake in postmenopausal women is 1,000–1,500 mg/day, and for vitamin D it is 400–800 IU/day (see **Table 7.4**). These values may vary, however, depending on age, ethnic group, nutrition status, and skeletal size.

Calcium appears to have little effect if given within the first 5 years of the menopause, when bone loss is predominantly due to estrogen withdrawal [13]. In prospective controlled trials, calcium supplements have been shown to reduce aging-associated bone loss by up to 50% (**Figure 7.1**) [13,14].

A retrospective case-control study has also shown a significant effect of calcium supplements on hip fracture risk [15], although data from controlled clinical trials have not yet been obtained. Calcium and vitamin D supplementation should be considered as a minimum treatment option in the frail and elderly, as supplementation with 1.2 g/day elemental calcium and 800 IU/day cholecalciferol has been shown to reduce the risk of hip fracture and other nonvertebral fractures in an elderly nursing-home population (**Figure 7.2**) [16]. Calcium and vitamin D should also be considered as an adjunct for other treatments.

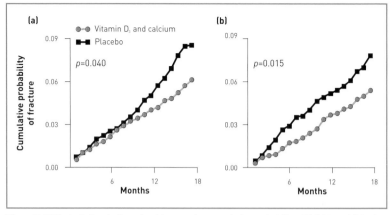

Figure 7.2 Effect of vitamin D$_3$ and calcium on the cumulative probability of **(a)** hip and **(b)** other nonvertebral fractures. Estimated by the life-table method and based on the length of time to the first fracture. Data from Chapuy et al [16].

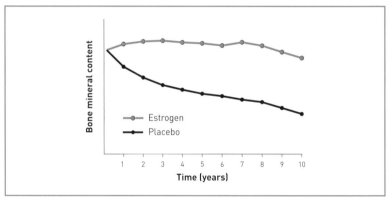

Figure 7.3 Bone mineral content in two groups of patients. Adapted from Lindsay et al [19].

Hormone replacement therapy

The association between osteoporosis and estrogen was first described by Fuller Albright in 1941 when he noted that 40 of 42 women with osteoporotic fractures were postmenopausal [17]. Subsequently, the associations between oophorectomy and accelerated bone loss and the beneficial effects of estrogen were observed (**Figures 7.3** and **7.4**) [18–20].

Bone mass has been positively associated with parity and use of the oral contraceptive, but results have not been consistent between studies. Hypo-estrogenic states that occur in anorexia nervosa and athletic amenorrhea are associated with low bone mass and increased fracture risk, although the

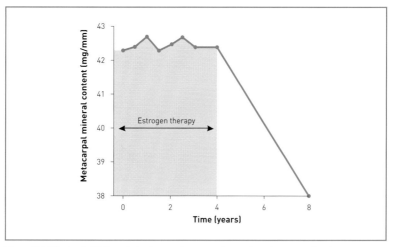

Figure 7.4 Effects of withdrawal of estrogen therapy on bone mineral content after 4 years of active treatment. Results are mean figures. Adapted from Lindsay et al [20].

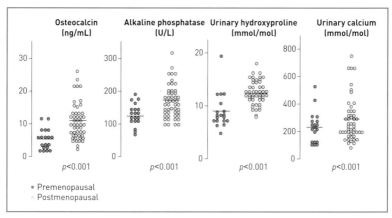

Figure 7.5 The effect of estrogen deficiency on biochemical indices of bone turnover. In postmenopausal women, bone formation (plasma osteocalcin and alkaline phosphatase) and bone resorption (urinary calcium and hydroxyproline) are increased compared with premenopausal women. Adapted from Christiansen and Lindsay [22].

pathogenic role of estrogen deficiency has not been definitely established. At the onset of the menopause, there is an increase in bone turnover, which results in net bone loss. Bone turnover can be assessed indirectly by measurement of biochemical markers of bone formation and resorption found in serum and urine (**Figure 7.5**), and studies show that treatment with hormone replacement therapy (HRT) causes these markers to return to premenopausal levels [21,22].

	CEE + MPA	CEE
Coronary heart disease	1.29 (1.02, 1.63)	0.91 (0.75, 1.12)
Stroke	1.41 (1.07, 1.85)	1.39 (1.10, 1.77)
Pulmonary embolism	2.13 (1.39, 3.25)	1.34 (0.87, 2.06)
Breast cancer	1.26 (1.00, 1.59)	0.77 (0.59, 1.01)
Colon cancer	0.63 (0.43, 0.92)	1.08 (0.75, 1.55)
Hip fracture	0.66 (0.45, 0.98)	0.61 (0.41, 0.91)
Death	0.98 (0.82, 1.18)	1.04 (0.88, 1.22)
Global index	1.15 (1.03, 1.28)	1.01 (0.91, 1.12)

Table 7.5 Data from the Women's Health Initiative showing the hazard ratios with 95% confidence intervals of various conditions in women treated with combined equine estrogen and medroxyprogesterone acetate (CEE + MPA) and those treated with CEE alone [28,29].

All estrogens appear to be capable of inhibiting bone loss, whether administered orally, transdermally, or subcutaneously. Adequate serum levels (>60 pg/mL) of estradiol are required to prevent this loss at the spine, and dose–response studies have indicated a minimum daily dose of 0.625 mg oral conjugated equine estrogens, 1 mg 17-β estradiol, or 15 mg ethinylestradiol. However, lower doses seem to be effective in elderly patients [23]. Higher doses may be needed to ensure that bone is not lost at the hip. Progestogens may also effectively reduce bone loss, particularly those derived from 19-nortestosterone [24,25].

Although HRT has long been known to reduce menopause-related bone loss, evidence for its fracture efficacy has been limited. Data from meta-analyses have demonstrated that HRT can reduce the risk of both vertebral and nonvertebral fractures [26,27]. These results have also been confirmed following the publication of the Women's Health Initiative (WHI), where treatment with HRT reduced clinical fractures in postmenopausal women [28]. The WHI study was a large (n=16,608), randomized, placebo-controlled, double-blind trial comparing the combination of conjugated equine estrogens (CEE) 0.625 mg daily plus medroxyprogesterone acetate 2.5 mg daily with placebo in postmenopausal women (aged 50–79 years) with an intact uterus. This trial was stopped 3 years early, after 5.2 years, because of unfavorable outcomes (**Table 7.5**). A further study was stopped early after 6.8 years. This looked at 10,739 postmenopausal women with a prior hysterectomy who were randomized to 0.625 mg/day CEE or placebo [29]. **Table 7.5** shows the hazard ratios from both studies.

Despite the beneficial effects on osteoporosis, treatment with HRT was associated with an increased risk of other diseases. Although the risks to an individual are small, HRT is no longer recommended as a first-choice therapy for the management of osteoporosis in postmenopausal women.

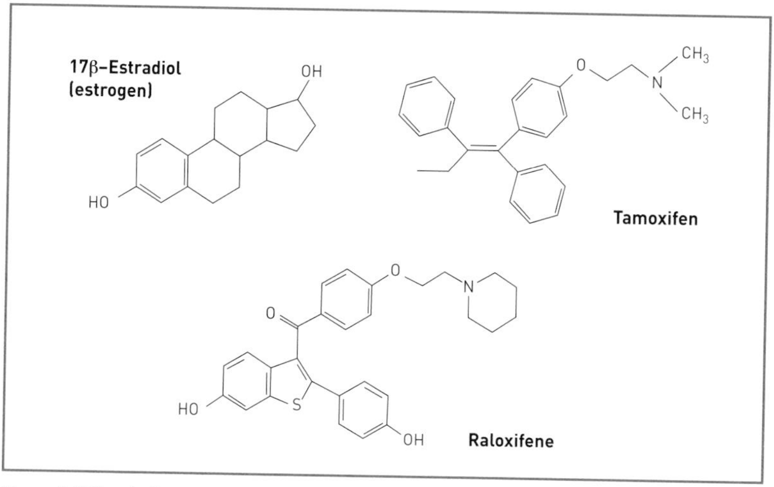

Figure 7.6 Chemical structures of estrogen, tamoxifen, and raloxifene.

It is currently recommended that HRT is considered for short-term use in the management of menopausal symptoms and that alternative agents are considered for the treatment of osteoporosis. Extended use of HRT may be advised where cessation of treatment causes a return of menopausal vasomotor symptoms and a poor quality of life. Such individuals should be counseled about the risks and benefits of treatment, and alternative options explored. They should undergo regular screening for breast cancer, and appropriate management of concurrent risk factors for vascular events would also be prudent.

Estrogen analogs

Tibolone is a synthetic estrogen, and its metabolites act on estrogen, progesterone, and androgen receptors. It has been demonstrated to prevent bone loss in early and late menopause [30,31], and is also used in the treatment of climacteric symptoms [32]. However, the effect of tibolone on reducing fracture risk has not been evaluated. Long-term studies are required to investigate its effect on the uterus and breast tissue, and on the frequency of cardiovascular disease: the Million Women Study has demonstrated that tibolone may be associated with an increased risk of breast cancer, with a relative risk of incident invasive breast cancer of 1.45 (95% confidence interval 1.25–1.67) [33]. The place of tibolone in the management of osteoporosis is therefore unclear.

Selective estrogen receptor modulators

Selective estrogen receptor modulators (SERMs) such as raloxifene and tamoxifen are designed to have tissue-specific effects, acting as either an estrogen agonist or antagonist (**Figure 7.6**). Currently, raloxifene is the only SERM licensed for the management of osteoporosis, although agents such as lasofoxifene are undergoing Phase III clinical trials.

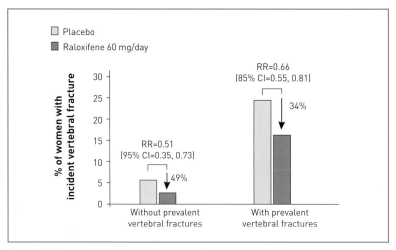

Figure 7.7 Effect of raloxifene in women with or without existing fractures. CI: confidence interval; RR: relative risk. Adapted from [59].

Raloxifene is a benzothiophene that acts as an agonist in bone and lipid metabolism, but as an antagonist in the breast and endometrium. In the Multiple Outcomes of Raloxifene Evaluation (MORE) study, 7,705 women with osteoporosis received raloxifene [34]. There was a significant reduction in vertebral fracture risk in both those with pre-existing vertebral fractures (reduction of 50%) and those without pre-existing vertebral fractures (reduction of 30%), although no effect was seen on nonvertebral fractures (**Figure 7.7**). These data therefore suggest that raloxifene should not be used in patients at high risk for hip fracture. It might be more suitable for women aged <70 years, although in the early postmenopausal years the incidence of menopausal vasomotor symptoms can be reduced. The MORE study also demonstrated that the frequency of breast cancer was lowered by 70% (**Figure 7.8**). This additional nonskeletal benefit may be important in aiding a decision on treatment.

Raloxifine has also been associated with an increased risk of DVT, similar to that seen with HRT. It is therefore contraindicated in patients with a history of thromboembolic disease. Raloxifine did not appear to be associated with an increased risk of cardiovascular events. In a secondary analysis of patients at high risk there was a suggestion of decreased cardiovascular risk [35]. This is being examined in ongoing studies.

Bisphosphonates
Bisphosphonates are synthetic analogs of pyrophosphate that bind to hydroxyapatite at sites of active bone remodeling. By inhibiting the action of osteoclasts, they reduce bone resorption. They contain a non-hydrolysable P-C-P bond and have two side chains: one that participates in binding to bone

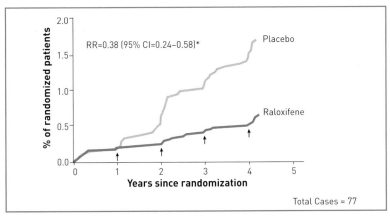

Figure 7.8 Effect of raloxifene on breast cancer incidence. Arrow denotes annual mammogram. CI: confidence interval; RR: relative risk. *p<0.001. Adapted from [60].

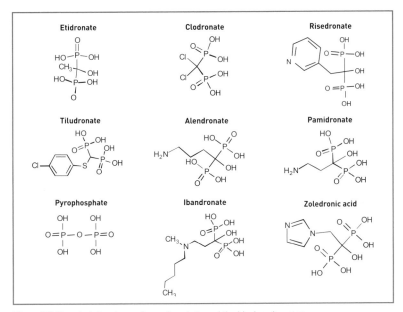

Figure 7.9 Chemical structures of pyrophosphate and the bisphosphonates.

and one that determines the pharmacologic properties of the drug (**Figure 7.9**). Absorption of an oral dose is less than 5% and subsequent uptake by bone is 30–40%, with the remainder undergoing renal excretion. Bisphosphonates have a short plasma half-life, but elimination from the skeleton is slow, with a half-life of several years in bone.

Etidronate was the first bisphosphonate to be developed and licensed for the management of osteoporosis. Treatment is given intermittently (400 mg/day for 2 weeks, repeated every 13 weeks). Two placebo-controlled studies have shown etidronate to increase spinal bone density by 4–5% during the first 2 years of treatment [36,37]. Despite certain limitations regarding the power of these two studies, the combined results suggest that this intermittent regimen of etidronate therapy is effective in reducing further vertebral fractures, and possibly accelerated bone loss, in patients with severe osteoporosis. The findings of a meta-analysis of controlled trials of etidronate over 1–4 years suggest a reduction in vertebral fracture risk, with a relative risk of 0.63 (95% confidence interval 0.44–0.92). No effect was seen for nonvertebral fractures [38].

Alendronate and risedronate are more potent inhibitors of bone resorption than etidronate, and have been shown to reduce fracture risk at all the clinically important sites, including the hip. In women with osteoporosis (as defined by BMD T-score below –2.5) and/or at least one vertebral fracture, treatment with alendronate was associated with a 50% reduction in fracture risk at the spine, wrist, and hip when compared with placebo [39]. Risedronate has also been shown to reduce the risk of vertebral [40] and nonvertebral [41] fracture. *Post-hoc* analyses of data from these studies have demonstrated that the reduction in vertebral fracture risk is seen within 6–12 months of starting treatment. The optimal treatment duration is not yet known, but one study has demonstrated that 10 years of treatment with alendronate is safe [42]. On the basis of changes in BMD and bone turnover markers, however, there may be no additional benefit to be gained beyond 5 years. The results of further studies with long-term data on BMD, bone turnover, and bone histology are awaited with interest. Compliance with therapy has been aided by once-weekly dosing, which is available for both risedronate (35 mg/week) and alendronate (70 mg/week). Intermittent dosing with oral ibandronate has also been shown to be effective in reducing risk of vertebral fracture [43] and a monthly dose may be available.

Oral bisphosphonates are generally well tolerated. However, in those with gastrointestinal intolerance or poor long-term compliance, intravenous treatment offers an alternative. Pamidronate infused every 3 months increases BMD at the spine and hip [44]. There are, however, no data on fractures with this intermittent dosing regimen. Zoledronate and ibandronate are two potent bisphosphonates that are undergoing Phase III clinical trials. Zoledronic acid, a cyclic nitrogen-containing third-generation bisphosphonate, is the most potent of the available bisphosphonates. A single 4 mg infusion of zoledronate has been shown to have effects on bone turnover for up to 12 months, with increases in BMD similar to those achieved with currently available oral bisphosphonates [45]. Studies are also examining a role for zoledronate treatment after hip fracture, in an attempt to reduce the risk of future fracture in an elderly, high-risk population. Bisphosphonates are now regarded as the treatment of choice for postmenopausal osteoporosis, due to proven efficacy and a good safety profile.

NICE has recently recommended bisphosphonates as first line therapy in patients with established osteoporosis [46].

Parathyroid hormone

Intermittent doses of human PTH given as daily subcutaneous injections have been shown to exert an anabolic effect, leading to increased osteoblast numbers and increases in bone formation. This contrasts with continuous exposure to PTH, which leads to increased bone resorption and a net decrease in trabecular bone volume. The (1-34) region of PTH has been demonstrated to be responsible for its anabolic action.

Currently, teriparatide (recombinant human PTH [1-34]) is the only formulation of PTH available for the management of osteoporosis. Treatment with teriparatide has been shown to increase BMD at the lumbar spine and femoral neck. It also reduces the risk of vertebral fractures by 65% and nonvertebral fractures overall by 53% [47]. The study was not powered to detect treatment effects at individual skeletal sites, and therefore there are no data on hip fracture reduction.

Teriparatide is the first of the bone-forming agents, and contrasts in its mode of action to the antiresorptive agents. Emerging data suggest that teriparatide has positive effects on both BMD and bone quality, and that these may play an important role in its ability to protect against fracture [48].

Teriparatide has been approved in Europe for the treatment of postmenopausal osteoporosis, with a treatment duration of 18 months. In the USA, treatment is licensed for 24 months and teriparatide is also available for use in men. There has been some interest that combined treatment with an anabolic agent and an anti-resorptive may provide additional benefit. Data published so far concerning combination treatments of PTH with alendronate have not shown any benefit [49,50]. Whether this is true of other bisphosphonates and SERMs is as yet unclear. After completion of the 18 month course of teriparatide it appears that fracture protection persists and to maximize this effect treatment should ideally be followed by an anti-resorptive agent [51].

Strontium ranelate

Strontium ranelate contains 2 atoms of stable strontium and an organic moiety (ranelic acid) **(Figure 7.10)**. In animal models it has been shown to both increase bone formation, by stimulation of preosteoblast replication leading to an increase in bone matrix synthesis by mature osteoblasts, and reduce bone formation, by inhibition of osteoclast activity and differentiation [52]. This has been confirmed in phase III human trials with increased bone specific alkaline phosphatase (a marker of bone formation) and decreased C-terminal peptide (a marker of bone resorption) [53].

In the SOTI (Spinal Osteoporosis Therapeutic Intervention) study of 1,649 postmenopausal women with established osteoporosis, a 49% reduction in risk

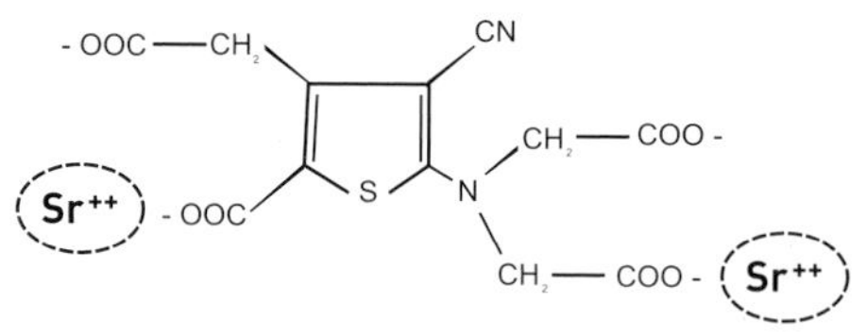

Figure 7.10 Chemical structure of strontium ranelate.

of new vertebral fracture was seen in the first year and a 41% reduction over 3 years, with a relative risk of 0.59 (95% confidence interval 0.48–0.73) [53]. This was accompanied by significant increases in BMD at the lumbar spine (14.4%) and femoral neck (8.3%) over 3 years. Bone histomorphometry has shown normal lamellar bone and normal mineralization.

In TROPOS (TReatment Of Peripheral Osteoporosis Study), 5,091 women aged ≥74 years (or 70–74 years with an additional risk factor) were involved in a double-blind, placebo controlled trial to look at nonvertebral fracture. There was a reduction in all nonvertebral fractures of 16% ($p=0.04$) after 3 years and a reduction of 19% ($p=0.031$) in major fragility fractures (hip, wrist, pelvis and sacrum, ribs and sternum, clavicle humerus) [54]. The study was not designed to look specifically at hip fracture; however, there was a nonsignificant decrease in risk of hip fracture of 15%. In a subgroup analysis of patients at high risk of hip fracture (aged ≥74 years and femoral neck T-score <–3) there was a risk reduction of 36% of hip fracture ($p=0.046$).

In general in this elderly population (combined mean age in TROPOS and SOTI =75 years) treatment was well tolerated and the most common adverse events were nausea and diarrhea.

Calcitonin

Calcitonin is an endogenous peptide of 32 amino acids that possesses antiosteoclastic activity. In clinical practice, four calcitonins (human, pig, salmon, and eel) have been used in studies of osteoporosis. Parenteral administration of calcitonin is either by intramuscular injection, suppository, or nasal spray.

Data for an effect of calcitonin on fracture risk are limited and mainly come from the Prevent Recurrence Of Osteoporotic Fractures (PROOF) study [55]. This was a 5-year, prospective, double-blind, randomized, placebo-controlled study of 1,255 postmenopausal women with osteoporosis. Data from this study demonstrated a reduction in vertebral fractures of 30% in individuals taking 200 IU of intranasal salmon calcitonin. There was, however, no effect on peripheral fractures. The study has subsequently been criticized for the following reasons: 60% of subjects in the study were lost to follow-up; doses of 100 IU and 400 IU had no effect on vertebral fracture risk; and there was no consistent effect on BMD and biochemical markers of bone turnover.

Although rarely used as a first-line treatment to prevent fractures, calcitonin has been shown to have analgesic properties that make it suitable for use in those with pain secondary to vertebral collapse, particularly in the acute state. The physiologic mechanisms underlying this action are poorly understood.

Other agents

Vitamin D analogs
Vitamin D analogs have been shown to reduce the rate of fracture in women with mild to moderate disease. In women >65 years of age with a previous fracture, addition of 1 mg of 1-α hydroxyvitamin D_3 (a pro-drug of 1,25[OH]D_3) and 300 mg elemental calcium daily for 1 year caused a significant decrease in the rate of new vertebral fractures [56]. A large randomized trial over 3 years in 432 women with osteoporosis (fewer than six vertebral fractures at study onset) also found that calcitriol 0.5 mg/day reduced the rate of new vertebral fractures compared with those treated with 1 g/day elemental calcium during the second (9.3 versus 25.0 fractures per 100 patient-years) and third (9.9 versus 31.5 fractures per 100 patient-years) years of the study [57]. Peripheral fractures were also reduced in the calcitriol group compared with the calcium-treated group (11 versus 24 fractures).

Toxicity is a concern with vitamin D analogs because of hypercalcemia and hypercalciuria, but the incidence of adverse events reported in the literature is low (<5%). These can be minimized by monitoring calcium intake, omitting calcium supplements, measuring urinary calcium excretion, increasing water intake, and administering vitamin D twice daily.

Fluoride
Fluoride was first recognized as a bone growth stimulator over 30 years ago, and sodium fluoride (NaF) and sodium monofluorophosphate (Na_2PO_4F) have been licensed for the treatment of osteoporosis in 10 European countries. The effect of fluoride on new fracture frequency is controversial and dependent on the dose and formulation of fluoride salt. Most studies have not shown increases in BMD at the cortical sites of the forearm or femoral neck, and there is concern that fluoride treatment may actually increase the risk for hip fracture. Currently, fluoride cannot be recommended for the treatment of postmenopausal osteoporosis.

Anabolic steroids
Anabolic steroids are derived from 19-norethisterone and are thought to be effective in preserving BMD, acting through a decrease in bone turnover. Their effect on bone mineral content can be explained in part by the increase in muscle mass and drop in body fat that accompanies treatment. However, the long-term

use of anabolic steroids in the treatment of osteoporosis will probably be limited by the presence of side-effects such as virilization, which are not negated by parenteral administration.

There is research interest in identifying drugs that will act as selective androgen receptor modulators (SARMs). These drugs will have tissue-specific effects, and it is hoped that a SARM will have positive effects on bone, with no evidence of virilization and no effect on lipid profiles.

Future agents

A growing number of new and novel treatments are emerging for the management of osteoporosis. With the discovery of the RANK ligand pathways there has been interest in using these as potential therapeutic targets. Preliminary data with a monoclonal antibody to RANKL suggest potent inhibition of bone resorption and increases in BMD with a twice yearly subcutaneous injection [58]. Phase III trials with fracture are ongoing and the results are awaited with interest.

Bone cells synthesize a large number of growth factors that enhance osteoblast proliferation. Various growth factors (eg, insulin-like growth factors 1 and 2, transforming growth factor-β) have been isolated, and are now available as potential treatment agents. Other compounds such as silicon derivatives are undergoing preclinical and clinical trials and might also soon be available for the treatment of established osteoporosis.

Conclusion

Osteoporosis and its related fractures is an important and major healthcare issue, with the incidence of fractures expected to increase significantly over the next 50 years. Drug treatment for this condition has evolved with an understanding of the disordered processes that underlie the development of low BMD and fracture. At present, a number of different drugs can be safely used with the expectation of preventing an initial or subsequent osteoporotic fracture.

HRT is no longer recommended as the first-choice treatment for postmenopausal osteoporosis, and bisphosphonates have now become the initial therapy of choice for most patients. SERMs such as raloxifene offer protection against vertebral fracture risk, with the additional benefit of a reduction in breast cancer risk. Agents such as teriparatide and strontium ranelate offer the potential to reverse, in part, the disease process. Newer biological agents also appear to offer an exciting therapeutic option. Exactly who will benefit from a particular therapy, the cost–benefit ratio of treatments, the duration of treatment, and the use of combinations of bone-forming and antiresorptive agents are the challenges for the next decade.

References

1. Consensus Development Conference. Prophylaxis and treatment of osteoporosis. *Osteoporos Int* 1991;1:114–17.
2. Dolan P, Torgerson D. The cost of treating osteoporotic fractures in the UK female population. *Osteoporos Int* 1998;8:611–17.
3. Melton LJ III, Chrischilles EA, Cooper C, et al. Perspective. how many people have osteoporosis? *J Bone Miner Res* 1992;7:1005–10.
4. Royal College of Physicans and Bone and Tooth Society. Osteoporosis – clinical guidelines for prevention and treatment. Update on pharmacologic interventions and an algorithm for management. London: Royal College of Physicians, 2000.
5. Law MR, Hackshaw AK. A meta-analysis of cigarette smoking, bone mineral density and risk of hip fracture: recognition of a major effect. *BMJ* 1997;315:841–6.
6. Taaffe DR, Duret C, Wheeler S, et al. Once weekly resistance exercise improves muscle strength and neuromuscular performance in older adults. *J Am Geriatr Soc* 1999;47:1208–14.
7. Meyer G, Warnke A, Bender R, et al. Effect on hip fractures of increased use of hip protectors in nursing homes: cluster randomized controlled trial. *BMJ* 2003;326:76.
8. Van Schoor NM, Deville WL, Bouter LM, et al. Acceptance and compliance with external hip protectors: a systemic review of the literature. *Osteoporos Int* 2002;13:917–24.
9. Lane JM, Giardi F, Kahn SN, et al. Preliminary outcomes of the first 226 consecutive kypoplasties for the fixation of painful osteoporotic vertebral compression fractures. *Osteoporos Int* 2000;11(Suppl 2):S206.
10. National Institute for Clinical Excellence. Percutaneous vertebroplasty. London: NICE, 2003. Available from: URL: http://www.nice.org.uk/page.aspx?o=85733 Accessed on April 25, 2005.
11. Kasperk C, Hillmeier J, Noldge G, et al. Treatment of painful vertebral fractures by kyphoplasty in patients with primary osteoporosis: a prospective nonrandomized controlled study. *J Bone Miner Res* 2005;20:604–12.
12. National Institute of Clinical Excellence. Balloon kyphoplasty for vertebral compression fracture. London: NICE, 2003. Available from: URL: http://www.nice.org.uk/page.aspx?o=91589 Accessed on April 25, 2005.
13. Dawson-Hughes B, Dallal GE, Krall EA, et al. A controlled trial of the effect of calcium supplementation on bone density in postmenopausal women. *N Engl J Med* 1990;323:878–83.
14. Reid IA, Ames RW, Evans MC, et al. Effect of calcium supplementation on bone loss in postmenopausal women. *N Engl J Med* 1993;328:460–4.
15. Kanis JA, Johnell O, Gullberg B, et al. Evidence for efficacy of drugs affecting bone metabolism in preventing hip fracture. *BMJ* 1992;305:1124–8.
16. Chapuy MC, Arlot ME, Delmas PD, et al. Effect of calcium and cholecalciferol treatment for three years on hip fracture in elderly women. *BMJ* 1994;308:1081–2.
17. Albright F, Smith PH, Richardson AM. Postmenopausal osteoporosis. *JAMA* 1941;116:2465–74.
18. Lindsay R, Tohme F. Estrogen treatment of patients with established postmenopausal osteoporosis. *Obstet Gynecol* 1990;76:290–5.
19. Lindsay R, Hart DM, Forrest C, et al. Prevention of spinal osteoporosis in oophorectomized women. *Lancet* 1980;ii:1151–4.
20. Lindsay R, Hart DM, MacLean A, et al. Bone response to termination of estrogen therapy. *Lancet* 1978;i:1325–7.
21. Uebelhart D, Schlemmer A, Johansen JS, et al. Effect of menopause and hormone replacement therapy on the urinary excretion of pyridinium cross-links. *J Clin Endocrinol Metab* 1991;72:367–73.
22. Christiansen C, Lindsay R. Estrogens, bone loss and preservation. *Osteoporosis Int* 1990;1:7–13.
23. Pors Nielsen S, Berenholdt O, Hermansen F, et al. Magnitude and pattern of skeletal response to long term continuous and cyclic sequential estrogen/progestin treatment. *Br J Obstet Gynaecol* 1994;101:319–24.
24. Lindsay R, Hart DM, Purdie D, et al. Comparative effects of estrogen and a progestogen on bone loss in postmenopausal women. *Clin Sci Mol Med* 1978;54:193–5.
25. Christiansen C, Riis BJ. 17beta-estradiol and continuous norethisterone: a unique treatment for established osteoporosis in elderly women. *J Clin Endocrinol Metab* 1990;71:836–41.
26. Torgerson DJ, Bell-Seyer SE. Hormone replacement therapy and prevention of vertebral fractures: a meta-analysis of randomized trials. *BMC Musculoskelet Disord* 2001;2:7.
27. Torgerson DJ, Bell-Seyer SE. Hormone replacement therapy and prevention of nonvertebral fractures: a meta-analysis of randomized trials. *JAMA* 2001;285:2891–7.
28. Rossouw JE, Anderson GL, Prentice RL, et al. Risks and benefits of estrogen plus progestin in healthy postmenopausal women: principal results from the women's health initiative randomized controlled trial. *JAMA* 2002;288:321–33.
29. Anderson GL, Limacher M, Assaf AR, et al. Effects of conjugated equine estrogen in postmenopausal women with hysterectomy: the Women's Health Initiative randomized controlled trial. *JAMA* 2004;291:1701–12.

30. Bjarnason NH, Bjarnason K, Haarbo J, et al. Tibolone: prevention of bone loss in late postmenopausal women. *J Clin Endocrinol Metab* 1996;81:2419–22.

31. Bernig B, Kuijk CV, Kuiper JW, et al. Effects of two doses of tibolone on trabecular and cortical bone loss in early postmenopausal women: a two-year randomized, placebo controlled study. *Bone* 1996;19:395–9.

32. Modelska K, Cummings S. Clinical review. Tibolone for postmenopausal women: Systemic review of randomized trials. *J Clin Endocrinol Metab* 2002;87:16–23.

33. Beral V. Million Women Study Collaborators. Breast cancer and hormone replacement therapy in the Million Women Study. *Lancet* 2003;362:419–27.

34. Ettinger B, Black DM, Mitlak BH, et al. Reduction of vertebral fracture risk in postmenopausal women with osteoporosis treated with raloxifene: results from a 3 year randomized clinical trial. *JAMA* 1999;282:637–45.

35. Barrett-Connor E, Grady D, Sashegyi A, et al. Raloxifene and cardiovascular events in osteoporotic postmenopausal women: four-year results from the MORE (Multiple Outcomes of Raloxifene Evaluation) randomized trial. *JAMA* 2002;287:847–57.

36. Storm T, Thamsborg G, Steiniche T, et al. Effect of intermittent cyclical etidronate therapy on bone mass and fracture rate in women with postmenopausal osteoporosis. *N Engl J Med* 1990;322:1265–71.

37. Harris ST, Watts NB, Jackson RD, et al. Four-year study of intermittent cyclic etidronate treatment of postmenopausal osteoporosis: three years of blinded therapy followed by one year of open therapy. *Am J Med* 1993;95:557–67.

38. Cranney A, Guyatt G, Krolicki N, et al. A meta-analysis of etidronate for the treatment of postmenopausal osteoporosis. *Osteoporos Int* 2001;12:140–51.

39. Black DM, Thompson DE, Bauer DC, et al. fracture risk reduction with aledronate in women with osteoporosis: the Fracture Intervention Trial. *J Clin Endocrinol Metab* 2000;85:4118–24.

40. Harris ST, Watts NB, Genant HK, et al. Effects of risedronate treatment on vertebral and nonvertebral fractures in women with postmenopausal osteoporosis: a randomized controlled trial. *JAMA* 1999;282:1344–52.

41. McClung MR, Geusens P, Miller PD, et al. Effect of risedronate on the risk of hip fracture in elderly women. *N Engl J Med* 2001;344:333–40.

42. Bone HG, Hosking D, Devogelaer JP, et al. Ten years' experience with alendronate for osteoporosis in postmenopausal women. *N Engl J Med*;2004:350:1189–99.

43. Chesnut CH, Skag A, Christiansen C, et al. Effects of oral ibandronate administered daily or intermittently in fracture risk in postmenopausal osteoporosis. *J Bone Miner Res* 2004;19:1241–9.

44. Reid IR, Wattie DJ, Evans MC, et al. Continuous therapy with pamidronate, a potent bisphosphonate, in postmenopausal osteoporosis. *J Clin Endocrinol Metab* 1994;79:1595–9.

45. Reid IR, Brown JP, Burckhardt P, et al. Intravenous zoledronic acid in postmenopausal women with low bone mineral density. *N Engl J Med* 2002;346:653–61.

46. National Institute of Clinical Excellence. Osteoporosis – secondary prevention. London: NICE, 2005. Available from: URL: http://www.nice.org.uk/page.aspx?0=241349 Accessed on April 25, 2005.

47. Neer RM, Arnaud CD, Zanchetta JR, et al. Effect of parathyroid hormone (1-34) on fractures and bone mineral density in postmenopausal women with osteoporosis. *N Engl J Med* 2001;344:1434–41.

48. Jiang Y, Zhao JJ, Mitlak BH, et al. Recombinant human parathyroid hormone (1–34) [teriparatide] improves both cortical and cancellous bone structure. *J Bone Miner Res* 2003;18:1932–41.

49. Black DM, Greenspan SL, Ensrud KE, et al. The effects of parathyroid hormone and alendronate alone or in combination in postmenopausal osteoporosis. *N Engl J Med* 2003;349:1207–15.

50. Finkelstein JS, Hayes A, Hunzelman JL, et al. The effects of parathyroid hormone, alendronate, or both in men with osteoporosis. *N Engl J Med* 2003;349:1216–26.

51. Lindsay R, Scheele WH, Neer R, et al. Sustained vertebral fracture risk reduction after withdrawal of teriparatide in postmenopausal women with osteoporosis. *Arch Intern Med* 2004;164:2024–30.

52. Marie PJ, Ammann P, Boivin B, et al. Mechanisms of action and therapeutic potential of strontium in bone. *Calcif Tissue Int* 2001;69:121–9.

53. Meunier PJ, Roux C, Seeman E, et al. The effects of strontium ranelate on risk of vertebral fracture in women with postmenopausal osteoporosis. *N Engl J Med* 2004;350:459–68.

54. Reginseter JY, Seeman E, De Vernejoul MC, et al. Strontium ranelate reduces the risk of nonvertebral fractures in postmenopausal women with osteoporosis: TROPOS study. *J Clin Endocrinol Metab* 2005 Feb 22; [Epub ahead of print].

55. Chesnut CH III, Silverman S, Andriano K, et al. A randomised trial of nasal spray salmon calcitonin in postmenopausal osteoporosis: the prevent recurrence of osteoporotic fracture study. *Am J Med* 2000;109:267–76.

56. Orimo H, Shiraki M, Hayashi Y, et al. Effects of 1 a-hydroxyvitamin D3 on lumbar bone mineral density and vertebral fractures in patients with postmenopausal osteoporosis. *Calcif Tissue Int* 1994;54:370–6.

57. Tilyard MW, Spears GF, Thomson J, et al. Treatment of postmenopausal osteoporosis with calcitriol or calcium. *N Engl J Med* 1992;326:357–62.

58. McClung MR, Lewiecki EM, Bolognese MA, et al. AMG 162 increases bone mineral density (BMD) within 1 month in postmenopausal women with low BMD. *J Bone Miner Res* 2004;19(Suppl 1):S20.

59. Eastell R, Adachi J, Harper K, et al. The effects of raloxifene on incident vertebral fractures in menopausal women with osteoporosis: 4-year results from the MORE trial. *J Bone Miner Res* 2000;15(Suppl 1):S229.

60. Cauley JA, Norton L, Lippman ME, et al. Continued breast cancer risk reduction in postmenopausal women treated with raloxifene: 4-year results from the MORE trial. *Breast Cancer Res Treat* 2001;65:125–134.

8

Osteoporosis in Men

Steve Tuck and Roger Francis

Introduction

Osteoporosis is a skeletal disorder characterized by compromised bone strength, predisposing a person to an increased risk of fracture. Although osteoporosis is widely considered to be a condition that predominantly affects women, up to 20% of symptomatic vertebral fractures, 25% of forearm fractures, and 30% of hip fractures occur in men [1]. Improved life expectancy and an increase in the age-specific incidence of fractures mean that the number of men presenting with these fractures is rising. Osteoporotic fractures are associated with excess mortality and substantial morbidity, which may be higher in men than in women. The annual cost of osteoporotic fractures in the UK was estimated at £942 million in 1998, of which 23% was due to fractures in men.

Epidemiology of fractures

The major osteoporotic fractures are those of the vertebral body and hip, but fractures of the forearm, humerus, tibia, pelvis, and ribs are also common. The incidence of most of these fractures rises steeply with age in both sexes, but the increase occurs earlier in women than in men, such that the fracture rate in elderly women is twice that of men of the same age (**Figure 8.1**) [2]. The lifetime risk of symptomatic fracture for a 50-year-old white man in the UK has been estimated to be 2% for the forearm, 2% for the vertebra, and 3% for the hip, compared with 13%, 11%, and 14%, respectively, for a 50-year-old woman.

Forearm fractures

Although the incidence of forearm fractures increases rapidly in women >50 years, there is little change in forearm fracture rate with age in men (**Figure 8.2**) [3]. This may reflect differences in the rate of falling with advancing age in men and women, as the risk of falls increases in middle age in women, but not until later life in men, when the outstretched arm is less likely to be used to break a fall. Although forearm fractures were not previously considered to be osteoporotic in men, a study showed that men with forearm fractures have a lower bone mineral density (BMD) than age-matched control subjects [4].

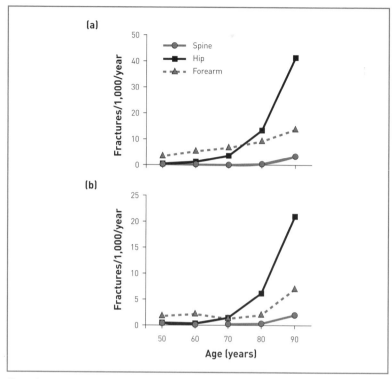

Figure 8.1 The incidence of forearm, symptomatic vertebral, and hip fractures in **(a)** women and **(b)** men from Cardiff, Wales [2].

Furthermore, men with forearm fractures have a 10.7- and 2.7-fold increased risk of subsequent vertebral and hip fracture, respectively [5].

Vertebral fractures

The incidence and prevalence of vertebral fractures is difficult to quantify, as many patients with this fracture do not come to medical attention. Data from Europe and the USA suggest that the prevalence of vertebral deformity may be higher in younger men than women, possibly due to trauma earlier in life [1]. There is also substantial geographic variation in the prevalence of vertebral deformity in men across Europe, with the highest rates in Scandinavian countries. The European Prospective Osteoporosis Study showed an increased incidence of morphometric vertebral fractures with age in both sexes (**Figure 8.3**), but the rates were higher in women than in men [6]. The only significant determinant of vertebral fracture incidence in men was body mass index (BMI), with reduced risk in those with a high BMI.

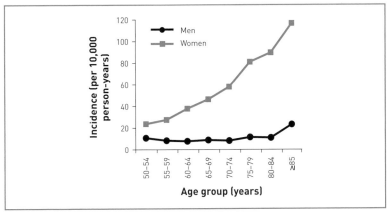

Figure 8.2 The incidence of forearm fractures in British men and women [3].

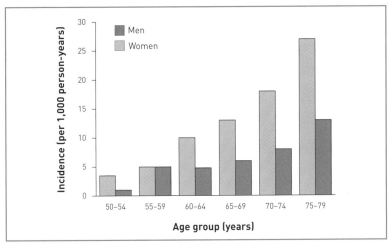

Figure 8.3 The incidence of morphometric vertebral fractures in men and women in the European Prospective Osteoporosis Study [6].

Hip fractures

The incidence of hip fractures increases with age in both sexes, in all geographical areas and ethnic groups. There is a greater difference in hip fracture incidence between ethnic groups and countries than between sexes, highlighting the potential importance of environmental, genetic, and lifestyle factors in the etiology of hip fractures. The highest incidence of hip fracture is in Scandinavia, with the lowest rates in Mediterranean countries [1].

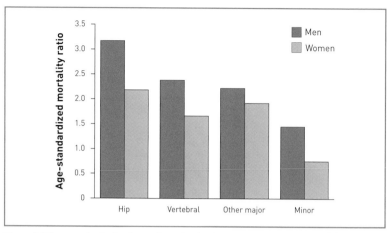

Figure 8.4 The age-standardized mortality ratio after fractures in men and women [7].

Mortality after osteoporotic fractures

There is increased mortality after all major fractures in both sexes, but the excess mortality is higher in men than in women (**Figure 8.4**). The standardized mortality ratio after a hip fracture is 3.17 in men and 2.18 in women, but the reason for the higher mortality in men remains uncertain [7]. Vertebral fractures are also associated with excess mortality in men compared with women, which may be due to a higher prevalence of coexisting conditions.

Morbidity after osteoporotic fractures

There is considerable disability after hip fracture in men, with only 21% living independently in the community a year later, whereas 26% receive home care and 53% live in an institution [1]. Although not all vertebral fractures come to medical attention, symptomatic fractures typically cause acute episodes of back pain, which usually settle after 6–8 weeks. Men with symptomatic vertebral fractures commonly complain of back pain, loss of height, and kyphosis, but also have significantly less energy, poorer sleep, more emotional problems, and impaired mobility than age-matched control subjects (**Figure 8.5**) [8].

Pathogenesis of osteoporosis

Bone mass at any age is determined by the peak bone mass, the age at which bone loss starts, and the rate at which it proceeds. Although peak bone mass is higher in men than in women, bone density at maturity is similar. The major determinants of peak bone density are genetic, but delayed puberty, poor dietary calcium intake, and lack of exercise during childhood and adolescence may lead to suboptimal peak bone mass, and therefore increase the risk of osteoporosis later in life [9].

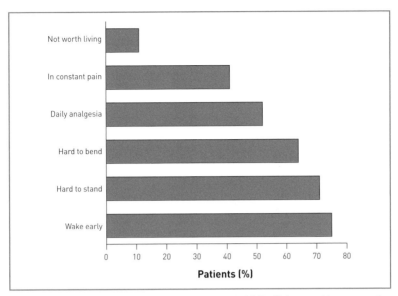

Figure 8.5 Responses to questions from the Nottingham Health Profile in men with symptomatic vertebral fractures [8].

Genetic factors

Genetic factors account for up to 80% of the variance in peak bone mass in both sexes. Men with a family history of osteoporosis have a lower than expected BMD and an increased risk of vertebral fractures. The major genes determining bone density and fracture risk in men remain uncertain, but candidate genes include those for collagen type IA1, the vitamin D receptor, vitamin D-binding protein, the estrogen receptor, and insulin-like growth factor (IGF)-I. Intrauterine development has also been implicated as a factor in the peak bone mass achieved, as there is an association between birth weight, childhood growth rate, and peak BMD [10].

Age-related factors

Bone loss starts between the ages of 35 and 50 years in men and women, and continues into old age in both sexes. The age-related decrease in circulating free testosterone, adrenal androgens, growth hormone, and IGF-I may contribute to the observed reduction in bone formation and continuing bone loss with age in men. Sex steroids play an important role in the maintenance of BMD in men, as demonstrated by the rapid bone loss seen after castration. Up to 20% of men with symptomatic vertebral fractures and 50% of men with hip fractures are hypogonadal. Nevertheless, it is now apparent that the actions of testosterone on the male skeleton may be mediated in part by aromatization to estradiol (**Figure 8.6**), such that estrogen deficiency contributes to age-related bone loss in men. Case reports have described osteoporosis in men with mutations in the

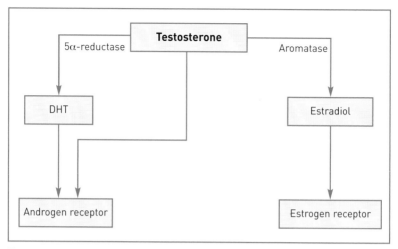

Figure 8.6 Schematic representation of the metabolism of sex steroids in men.
DHT: dihydrotestosterone.

estrogen receptor or aromatase genes. Studies have shown that BMD and the prevalence of vertebral fractures in men are related to serum estradiol (**Figure 8.7**), but not to serum testosterone [11,12].

Other factors

A number of other factors have been implicated in bone loss in men [9], including:

- low BMI
- smoking
- physical inactivity
- heredity
- alcohol consumption
- poor dietary calcium
- impaired vitamin D production and metabolism
- secondary hyperparathyroidism

The development of osteoporosis may be accelerated by underlying secondary causes of bone loss, which are found in over 50% of men presenting with symptomatic vertebral crush fractures (**Figure 8.8**) [8,13]. Case-control studies of hip fractures in men have shown an increased risk of fracture with disorders associated with secondary osteoporosis [14,15]. The major secondary causes of osteoporosis in men are listed in **Table 8.1**.

A case-control study from the Mayo Clinic, USA, investigated 105 men with vertebral fractures and 105 age-matched control subjects with Paget's disease of

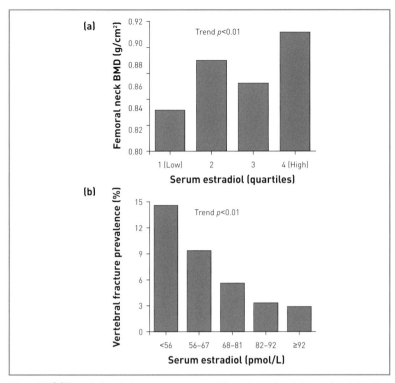

Figure 8.7 (a) The relationship between serum estradiol and femoral neck bone mineral density (BMD) in men [11]. **(b)** The relationship between serum estradiol and the prevalence of vertebral fractures [12].

bone. This showed a significantly increased relative risk of vertebral fractures with smoking, alcohol consumption, and underlying secondary causes of osteoporosis, while the risk was reduced in the presence of obesity [16]. A subsequent case-control study from Newcastle upon Tyne, UK, demonstrated an increased risk of vertebral fractures with oral steroid therapy, anticonvulsant treatment, smoking, alcohol intake of >20 units/week, physical inactivity, and family history (**Figure 8.9**) [8].

Pathogenesis of fractures

The risk of fracture is determined by skeletal and nonskeletal risk factors. The skeletal risk factors include BMD, bone turnover, trabecular architecture, bone size, skeletal geometry, and bone quality, whereas nonskeletal risk factors include postural instability and propensity for falling. There is an inverse relationship between BMD and the incidence of vertebral and hip fractures in men (**Figure 8.10**), which is similar to that observed in women [17,18].

Major causes with strong evidence	
Hypogonadism	Oral glucocorticoids
Alcoholism	Transplantation
Other causes	
Endocrine	Drugs
• Hyperparathyroidism	• Anticonvulsants
• Thyrotoxicosis	• Warfarin
Gastrointestinal	Idiopathic hypercalciuria
• Celiac disease	Malignancy
• Inflammatory bowel disease	Chemotherapy
• Liver cirrhosis	
• Gastric surgery	
• Bowel resection	

Table 8.1 Causes of secondary osteoporosis in men.

Case-control studies show that men with distal forearm, symptomatic vertebral, and hip fractures have lower BMD than age-matched control subjects [4,8,19]. In men with vertebral and hip fractures, the greatest reduction in BMD is seen at the lumbar spine and femoral neck, respectively (**Figure 8.11**).

There is growing evidence that men with fractures not only have a lower BMD, but also a smaller skeletal size than age- and sex-matched control subjects. A study in men with vertebral fractures demonstrated a lower BMD at all sites compared with control subjects, but also showed that the fracture group had a smaller area and width of the lumbar vertebrae [20]. There was no difference in vertebral height, suggesting that lack of periosteal apposition was the problem, rather than a failure of longitudinal growth.

Skeletal geometry also plays a role in determining fracture risk. This has been most extensively studied in women at the hip, in terms of hip axis length (HAL), femoral neck axis length, neck shaft angle (NSA), femoral neck width, and pelvic size. The role of all of these factors as independent predictors of hip fracture risk is controversial in both sexes, with studies giving conflicting results. Men with hip fractures have a wider pelvis, shorter HAL, wider femoral necks, and larger NSAs than male control subjects [21]. A larger study found that a standard deviation increase in NSA or femoral neck width approximately doubled the risk of hip fracture in men, but there was no association with HAL [22].

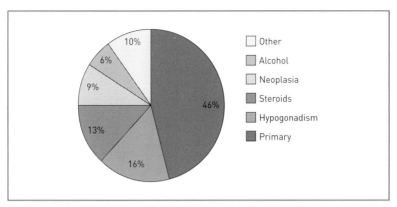

Figure 8.8 The major causes of secondary osteoporosis in a group of men with symptomatic vertebral fractures presenting to the Bone Clinic in Newcastle upon Tyne, UK [13].

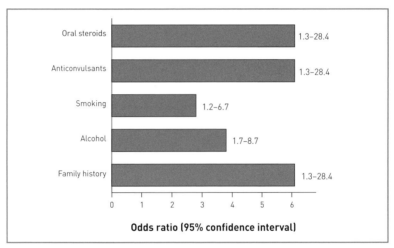

Figure 8.9 Significant risk factors for symptomatic vertebral fractures identified in a case-control study from Newcastle upon Tyne, UK [8].

The importance of nonskeletal risk factors for fracture is demonstrated by the greater risk of hip fracture in men with conditions that are associated with an increased risk of falling, such as hemiparesis, Parkinson's disease, dementia, vertigo, alcoholism, and blindness [14]. A prospective study from Australia also showed a higher risk of hip fracture in men with low hip BMD, quadriceps weakness, increased body sway, falls in the past year, previous fractures, low body weight, and short stature [23].

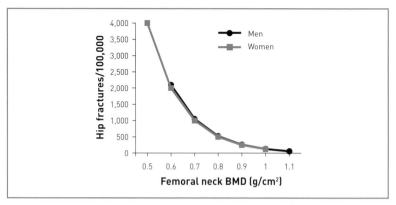

Figure 8.10 The relationship between femoral neck bone mineral density (BMD) and the incidence of hip fractures in 80-year-old men and women in the Rotterdam Study, The Netherlands [17].

Diagnosis of osteoporosis

Until recently, the diagnosis of osteoporosis in men was based on the development of fractures after minimal trauma. The introduction of dual-energy X-ray absorptiometry (DXA) bone density measurement has stimulated interest in the diagnosis of osteoporosis before fractures occur. The World Health Organization (WHO) has defined osteoporosis as a BMD ≥2.5 standard deviations below the mean value for young adults (T-score less than –2.5), but this has only been established for women.

Although the reference ranges for BMD measurements in men are derived from a smaller sample size than in women, there is a similar inverse relationship between absolute BMD and the incidence of vertebral and hip fractures in both sexes [17,18]. This indicates that the same threshold value of absolute BMD could be used for the diagnosis of osteoporosis in men and women. A T-score of –2.5 in women would therefore be equivalent to a T-score of –2.8 in men, calculated using gender-specific normative data. The prevalence of osteoporosis in men using this diagnostic threshold is too low, whereas the prevalence of a T-score less than –2.5 at the hip, spine, or forearm in men >50 years is broadly comparable to the lifetime risk of fractures at these sites [24]. This suggests that the WHO criteria may be applicable for the diagnosis of osteoporosis in both men and women.

Although only approximately 50% of men with apparently low-trauma vertebral fractures have densitometric evidence of osteoporosis at the lumbar spine or femoral neck, a further 40% have osteopenia [8]. We therefore suggest that treatment for osteoporosis should be considered in men with low-trauma vertebral fractures and evidence of osteoporosis or osteopenia at the lumbar spine or femoral neck, whereas the possibility of unrecognized antecedent trauma should be explored in those with normal BMD measurements.

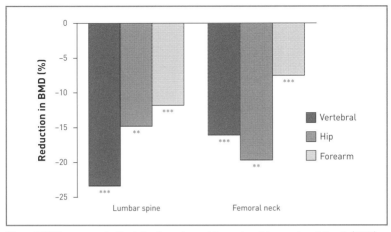

Figure 8.11 The mean reduction in lumbar spine and femoral neck bone mineral density (BMD) in men with forearm [4], symptomatic vertebral [8], and hip [19] fractures compared with age-matched male control subjects. The statistical significance is indicated (**$p<0.01$, ***$p<0.001$).

Investigation of osteoporosis

Secondary causes of osteoporosis should be sought by taking a careful history, physical examination, and conducting appropriate investigation (**Table 8.2**). Serum testosterone should be measured in a morning urine sample, because of the diurnal variation in circulating concentration. A recent hip fracture may alter the hypothalamic–pituitary–gonadal axis, as well as increasing alkaline phosphatase levels, so investigations for secondary osteoporosis should be performed after the patient has recovered from the fracture and subsequent surgery.

Prostate-specific antigen should also be measured in men with vertebral fractures and symptoms of prostatism or evidence of sclerosis on X-rays. In elderly men with osteoporosis, serum 25-hydroxyvitamin D and intact parathyroid hormone (PTH) measurements can be used to exclude vitamin D insufficiency and secondary hyperparathyroidism. These investigations are probably unnecessary if calcium and vitamin D supplementation is planned.

These investigations are usually normal in men with idiopathic osteoporosis, apart from a transient rise in serum alkaline phosphatase after fracture. The most frequently encountered causes of secondary osteoporosis in men are oral steroid therapy, hypogonadism, alcohol abuse, myeloma, and skeletal metastases. In men with severe unexplained osteoporosis, it may be worth considering 24-hour urine calcium estimation to identify hypercalciuria, 24-hour urine cortisol to exclude Cushing's syndrome, and antiendomysial antibodies to look for celiac disease.

Investigation	Finding	Possible cause
Full blood count	Anemia	Neoplasia or malabsorption
	Macrocytosis	Alcohol abuse or malabsorption
ESR	Raised ESR	Neoplasia
Biochemical profile	Hypercalcemia	Hyperparathyroidism or neoplasia
	Abnormal liver function	Alcohol abuse or liver disease
	Persistently high AP	Skeletal metastases
Thyroid function tests	Suppressed TSH; high T$_4$ or T$_3$	Hyperthyroidism
Serum and urine immunoelectrophoresis (vertebral fractures)	Paraprotein band	Myeloma
Testosterone, SHBG, LH, FSH	Low testosterone or free testosterone index with raised or low gonadotrophins	Hypergonadotrophic hypogonadism / Hypogonadism
Prostate-specific antigen	Markedly raised levels	Skeletal metastases from prostate cancer

Table 8.2 Investigations for secondary osteoporosis in men. AP: alkaline phosphatase; ESR: erythrocyte sedimentation rate; FSH: follicle-stimulating hormone; LH: luteinizing hormone; SHBG: sex hormone-binding globulin; T$_3$: tri-iodothyronine; T$_4$: normal thyroxine; TSH: thyroid-stimulating hormone.

Management of osteoporosis

The management of osteoporosis should include symptom relief, lifestyle measures to prevent bone loss and decrease the risk of falls, and specific treatment to increase BMD and reduce the incidence of fractures. All patients should be offered analgesia appropriate for the severity of their pain. Transcutaneous electrical nerve stimulation (TENS) is also of value in some patients with vertebral fractures. Advice from a physiotherapist may help to maintain mobility and prevent falls, as might occupational therapy assessment. Advice and support is also available from self-help groups such as the National Osteoporosis Society in the UK (www.nos.org.uk) or the National Osteoporosis Foundation in the USA (www.nof.org).

Men with osteoporosis should be given advice on lifestyle measures to decrease bone loss, including a balanced diet rich in calcium, weight-bearing exercise, smoking cessation, moderation of alcohol intake, and maintenance of regular exposure to sunlight. Where there is a history of recurrent falls, falls assessment and multifactorial intervention strategies may decrease future risk. Hip protectors potentially decrease the risk of hip fractures in frail elderly patients after recurrent falls, although compliance with their use is poor.

Treatment of osteoporosis

Any underlying secondary cause of osteoporosis should be treated if possible, as specific treatment of underlying conditions such as hyperthyroidism, hypogonadism, and hyperparathyroidism can increase bone density by 10–20%. There are a number of therapeutic options for idiopathic osteoporosis in men, including bisphosphonates, calcitonin, anabolic steroids, androgens, teriparatide, calcium and vitamin D supplementation, calcitriol, and fluoride salts.

Bisphosphonates

Bisphosphonates have become the treatment of choice for most men with osteoporosis. Observational studies in men with idiopathic and secondary osteoporosis suggest that intermittent cyclical etidronate therapy increases BMD at the lumbar spine by 5–10%, with smaller increases at the hip. In an uncontrolled study of 42 men with vertebral fractures, cyclical etidronate increased spine BMD by 3% annually, while hip bone density showed a nonsignificant rise of 0.7% per year [25]. It would therefore appear that cyclical etidronate has comparable effects on bone density in men and women, although the effect on fracture incidence in men remains unclear.

A recent randomized, controlled trial (RCT) compared the effect of 2 years' treatment with alendronate and placebo in 241 men with osteoporosis aged 31–87 years, 36% of whom were hypogonadal [26]. This showed a significant improvement in lumbar spine and femoral neck BMD with alendronate (**Figure 8.12**), with similar BMD increases in eugonadal and hypogonadal men. There was also a significant reduction in vertebral fracture incidence and decrease in height loss with alendronate. Similar results were reported in another RCT in 134 men with primary osteoporosis [27]. The daily preparation of alendronate has now been licensed in the USA and UK for the treatment of osteoporosis in men. There is no reason to think that the 70 mg weekly preparation would not be equally effective, and many patients find the weekly preparation more convenient.

In a 3-year RCT in 677 men and women with osteoporosis and at least one vertebral fracture, 84 men were randomized to receive clodronate or placebo [28]. Interim analysis at 1 year showed a significant increase in lumbar spine and total hip BMD with clodronate compared with placebo, with similar changes in men and women. There was also an overall reduction in vertebral fracture incidence with clodronate. It would therefore appear likely that bisphosphonates are equally effective in the management of men and women with osteoporosis. Although there are no published studies on the effect of risedronate in men with idiopathic osteoporosis, there is no reason to suspect that it would be ineffective,

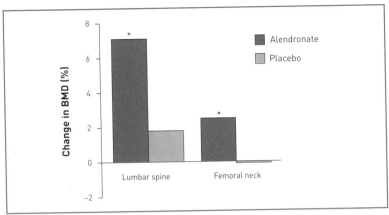

Figure 8.12 The change in lumbar spine and femoral neck bone mineral density (BMD) in men with osteoporosis treated with alendronate or placebo [26]. The statistical significance between the two groups is indicated, *$p<0.001$.

particularly as it has been shown to be beneficial in men and women with glucocorticoid-induced osteoporosis.

Calcitonin

A small study in 28 men with osteoporosis showed that nasal calcitonin, 200 IU daily for 12 months, increased lumbar spine BMD by 4.7% compared with control subjects (**Figure 8.13**), but resulted in no significant change in BMD at the proximal femur [29]. Calcitonin may also be useful in the management of patients with acute vertebral fracture. An RCT in 32 men and 68 women with acute vertebral fracture showed that intranasal calcitonin, 200 IU daily for 28 days, was more effective than placebo at decreasing pain and improving mobility [30].

Anabolic steroids

Although agents such as nandrolone decanoate transiently increase bone density in men with osteoporosis, the benefit may be lost in the longer term. This might be due to suppression of the pituitary–gonadal axis, with a consequent reduction in endogenous sex hormone production [31]. Such treatment may also lead to abnormalities in liver function. Anabolic steroids should therefore be regarded as an experimental treatment.

Androgens

In addition to improving BMD in men with hypogonadal osteoporosis [32], testosterone may increase spine BMD in eugonadal men with vertebral fractures (**Figure 8.14**). An uncontrolled study of testosterone treatment in 21 eugonadal men with vertebral osteoporosis showed a significant increase in spine BMD of 5% in 6 months, but no change in hip BMD was seen [33]. During this time, there was a 48% increase in serum testosterone and a 22% reduction in sex

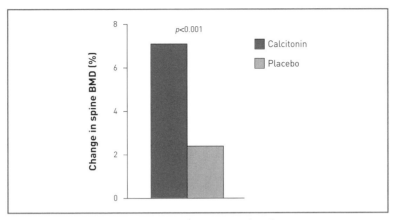

Figure 8.13 The change in lumbar spine bone mineral density (BMD) in men with osteoporosis treated with calcitonin or placebo [29]. The statistical significance between the two groups is indicated.

hormone-binding globulin, leading to an 88% increase in free androgen index. Serum estradiol also increased by 41%. The biochemical markers of bone turnover showed a reduction in bone formation and resorption (**Figure 8.15**). Analysis of the changes in BMD and sex steroid concentrations showed a closer relationship between the changes in BMD and serum estradiol than with serum testosterone. An RCT in 15 men on long-term glucocorticoid treatment showed an increase in spine BMD of 5% after 12 months' treatment with testosterone, while no change was observed during the control period of 12 months' observation [34]. Side-effect and cardiovascular risk factor profiles were acceptable in these small studies, and androgen treatment is to be more fully explored in a multicenter RCT. Until the results of such studies are available, this treatment should also be regarded as experimental.

Teriparatide

Another anabolic agent that may be useful in treating osteoporosis in men is teriparatide (recombinant human parathyroid hormone [rhPTH(1-34)]). PTH stimulates both bone formation and resorption, leading to increased or decreased BMD, depending on the mode of administration. Continuous infusion causes persistent elevation of PTH and results in greater resorption than formation, leading to bone loss. By contrast, daily injections of PTH lead to only transient peaks in serum PTH, resulting in greater bone formation and an increase in BMD.

In postmenopausal women with prior vertebral fractures, teriparatide increases BMD and reduces both vertebral and nonvertebral fractures [35]. In a small study of subcutaneous rhPTH(1-34) treatment (400 IU daily in 23 men aged 30–68 years), BMD increased by 13.5% in the lumbar spine and by 2.9% at the

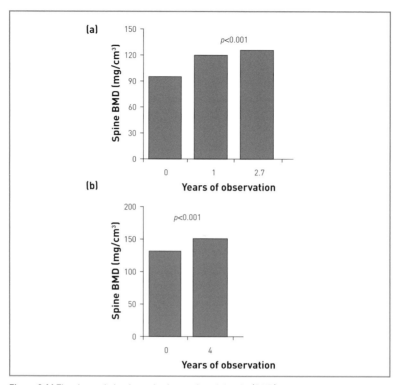

Figure 8.14 The change in lumbar spine bone mineral density (BMD) measured by quantitative computerized tomography in hypogonadal men on testosterone replacement therapy [32]. **(a)** The results in men who were previously untreated; **(b)** the results in men already on testosterone treatment. The statistical significance of changes from the baseline value is indicated.

femoral neck over 18 months (**Figure 8.16**) [36]. Another study in 437 osteoporotic men showed significant increases in lumbar spine and femoral neck BMD after a median of 11 months' treatment with subcutaneous teriparatide (20 and 40 µg daily) (**Figure 8.17**) [37]. Side-effects of teriparatide include nausea, headache, and transient mild hypercalcemia, but these were reported less commonly with the 20 µg dose. Teriparatide became available in the UK and USA from late 2003, with a recommended dose of 20 µg daily for an 18-month course of treatment.

Calcium and vitamin D

The role of calcium and vitamin D supplementation in the management of osteoporosis in men remains unclear. In an RCT of 86 healthy men aged 30–87 years, supplementation with 1,000 mg of calcium and 1,000 IU of vitamin D daily had no effect on bone loss from the forearm or spine [38]. By contrast, a US RCT in 389 older men and women (mean age 70 years) who were living at home demonstrated that 700 IU vitamin D_3 and 500 mg elemental calcium daily

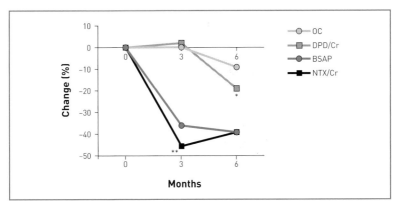

Figure 8.15 The change in the biochemical markers of bone formation and bone resorption in an observational study of eugonadal men with osteoporosis treated with testosterone [33]. The statistical significance of changes from the baseline value is indicated (*$p<0.05$, **$p<0.01$). BSAP: bone-specific alkaline phosphatase; Cr: creatinine; DPD: urine deoxypyridinoline; NTX: urine N-terminal telopeptide; OC: osteocalcin.

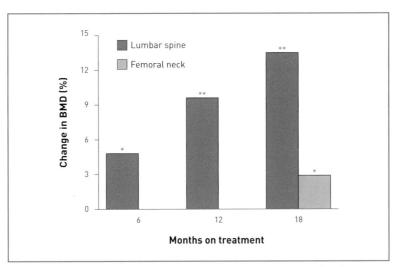

Figure 8.16 The change in lumbar spine and femoral neck bone mineral density (BMD) on treatment with subcutaneous recombinant human parathyroid hormone (rhPTH), 400 IU daily compared with placebo in men with osteoporosis [36]. The statistical significance of differences from the placebo group is indicated (*$p<0.05$, **$p<0.01$).

had a modest beneficial effect on BMD, and decreased the incidence of nonvertebral fractures [39]. Subgroup analysis of the results for the men in this study showed a significant improvement in BMD with calcium and vitamin D,

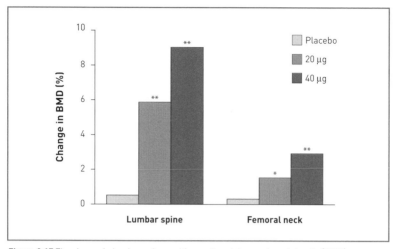

Figure 8.17 The change in lumbar spine and femoral neck bone mineral density (BMD) on treatment with subcutaneous teriparatide 20 µg and 40 µg daily or placebo injections in men with osteoporosis. The statistical significance of differences from the placebo group is indicated (*$p<0.05$, **$p<0.001$).

but no reduction in fractures was demonstrated. A recent study of oral vitamin D_3, 100,000 IU every 4 months, in 2,037 men and 649 women aged 65–85 years, living in the community, showed an overall 22% reduction in fracture risk [40]. There was no significant reduction in fractures at any specific site or in either gender alone. In the absence of more conclusive studies, it seems reasonable to recommend calcium and vitamin D supplementation in frail, elderly men, who are likely to have vitamin D deficiency and secondary hyperparathyroidism. Calcium and vitamin D may also be used as an adjunct to other treatments in men with established osteoporosis.

Calcitriol
Calcitriol is a synthetic form of 1,25 dihydroxyvitamin D, the hormonally active metabolite of vitamin D. Calcitriol promotes calcium absorption from the bowel and may stimulate osteoblastic new bone formation. In a small RCT in 41 men with idiopathic osteoporosis, there was no difference in the change in spine or femoral neck BMD between those treated with calcitriol and the control group taking calcium supplements [41].

Fluoride salts
Some clinical trials of fluoride have included men, but it is difficult to ascertain whether responses were in any way gender-specific. A German RCT showed that low-dose intermittent monofluorophosphate and calcium increases bone density and decreases the risk of vertebral fractures in men with osteoporosis [42].

Monitoring of treatment

Approximately 10–15% of patients fail to respond to treatment [43]. Therefore, at least one repeat DXA scan is recommended to confirm treatment response. This is usually best done after at least 2 years of treatment, as it takes this long for the response to antiresorptive agents to exceed the least significant change in BMD. Furthermore, the BMD may fall during the first year of treatment, only to subsequently gain in the second year – a phenomenon known as regression to the mean [44].

The use of BMD to assess response has disadvantages. It takes 2 years before a lack of response is noted, and the use of the spine can be affected by degenerative changes, especially in patients >65 years and in younger men with manual occupations. An alternative is to use bone turnover markers, which have a maximum suppression in the order of 50% within 3 months of starting therapy [45]. This would allow earlier identification of nonresponders. However, these can be difficult to collect, tend to be very variable, are influenced by many factors, and it is not known whether changes in bone turnover markers reflect a reduction in fracture risk. In light of these difficulties, it is currently recommended that their use be confined to specialist centers and research.

Conclusion

Osteoporotic fractures are a major public health problem in both men and women. Further work is required to clarify the pathogenesis of osteoporosis and fractures in men, and to develop diagnostic criteria for this. More studies are also needed to establish the most effective treatment for osteoporosis in men. Underlying secondary causes of osteoporosis should be treated where possible, and bisphosphonates are probably the treatment of choice. Calcium and vitamin D supplements may be useful in frail, elderly men with osteoporosis, who are likely to have vitamin D deficiency and secondary hyperparathyroidism. New, exciting anabolic agents such as teriparatide should further enhance the treatment of this disabling condition.

References

1. Pande I, Francis RM. Osteoporosis in men. *Best Pract Res Clin Rheumatol* 2001;15:415–27.
2. Johansen A, Evans RJ, Stone MD, et al. Fracture incidence in England and Wales: A study based on the population of Cardiff. *Injury* 1997;28:655–60.
3. O'Neill TW, Cooper C, Finn JD, et al. Incidence of distal forearm fracture in British men and women. *Osteoporos Int* 2001;12:555–8.
4. Tuck SP, Raj N, Summers GD. Is distal forearm fracture in men due to osteoporosis? *Osteoporos Int* 2002;13:630–6.
5. Cuddihy MT, Gabriel SE, Crowson CS, et al. Forearm fractures as predictors of subsequent osteoporotic fracture. *Osteoporos Int* 1999;9:469–75.
6. Roy DK, O'Neill TW, Finn JD, et al. Determinants of incident vertebral fracture in men and women: results for the European Prospective Osteoporosis Study (EPOS). *Osteoporos Int* 2003;14:19–26.
7. Center JR, Nguyen TV, Schneider D, et al. Mortality after all major types of fracture in men and women: an observational study. *Lancet* 1999;353:878–82.

8. Scane AC, Francis RM, Sutcliffe AM, et al. Case-control study of the pathogenesis and sequelae of symptomatic vertebral fractures in men. *Osteoporos Int* 1999;9:91–7.

9. Scane AC, Francis RM. Risk factors for osteoporosis in men. *Clin Endocrinol* 1993;38:15–16.

10. Cooper C, Walker-Bone K, Arden N, et al. Novel insights into the pathogenesis of osteoporosis: the role of intrauterine programming. *Rheumatology* 2000;39:1312–15.

11. Amin S, Zhang Y, Sawin CT, et al. Association of hypogonadism and estradiol levels with bone mineral density in elderly men from the Framingham Study. *Ann Intern Med* 2000;133:951–63.

12. Barrett-Conner E, Mueller JE, von Muhlen DG, et al. Low levels of estradiol are associated with vertebral fractures in older men, but not women: the Rancho Bernardo Study. *J Clin Endocrinol Metab* 2000;85:219–23.

13. Baillie SP, Davison CE, Johnson FJ, et al. Pathogenesis of vertebral crush fractures in men. *Age Ageing* 1992;21:139–41.

14. Poor G, Atkinson EJ, O'Fallon WM, et al. Predictors of hip fractures in elderly men. *J Bone Miner Res* 1995;10:1900–7.

15. Stanley HL, Schmitt BP, Poses RM, et al. Does hypogonadism contribute to the occurrence of a minimal trauma hip fracture in elderly men? *J Am Geriatr Soc* 1991;39:766–71.

16. Seeman E, Melton LJ III, O'Fallon WM, et al. Risk factors for spinal osteoporosis in men. *Am J Med* 1983;75:977–83.

17. De Laet CE, Van Hout BA, Burger H, et al. Bone density and risk of hip fracture in men and women: cross-sectional analysis. *BMJ* 1997;315:221–5.

18. Van der Klift M, De Laet CE, McCloskey EV, et al. The incidence of vertebral fractures in men and women: the Rotterdam Study. *J Bone Miner Res* 2002;17:1051–6.

19. Pande I, O'Neill TW, Pritchard C, et al. Bone mineral density, hip axis length and risk of hip fractures in men: results from the Cornwall Hip Fracture Study. *Osteoporos Int* 2000;11:866–70.

20. Vega E, Ghiringhelli G, Mautalen C, et al. Bone mineral density and bone size in men with primary osteoporosis and vertebral fractures. *Calcif Tissue Int* 1998;62:465–9.

21. Karlsson KM, Sernbo I, Obrant KJ, et al. Femoral neck geometry and radiographic signs of osteoporosis as predictors of hip fracture. *Bone* 1996;18:327–30.

22. Alonso CG, Curiel MD, Carranza FH, et al. Femoral bone mineral density, neck-shaft angle and mean femoral neck width as predictors of hip fracture in men and women. *Osteoporos Int* 2000;11:714–20.

23. Nguyen TV, Eisman JA, Kelly PJ, et al. Risk factors for osteoporotic fractures in elderly men. *Am J Epidemiol* 1996;144:255–63.

24. Melton LJ III, Atkinson EJ, O'Connor MK, et al. Bone density and fracture risk in men. *J Bone Miner Res* 1998;13:1915–23.

25. Anderson FH, Francis RM, Bishop JC, et al. Effect of intermittent cyclical disodium etidronate therapy on bone mineral density in men with vertebral fractures. *Age Ageing* 1997;26:359–65.

26. Orwoll E, Ettinger M, Weiss S, et al. Alendronate treatment of osteoporosis in men. *N Engl J Med* 2000;343:604–10.

27. Ringe JD, Faber H, Dorst A. Alendronate treatment of established primary osteoporosis in men: results of a 2 year prospective study. *J Clin Endocrinol Metab* 2001;86:5252–5.

28. McCloskey E, Selby P, Davies M, et al. Clodronate decreases vertebral fracture incidence in men and women with established osteoporosis. *Calcif Tissue Int* 1999;64(Suppl 1):S82.

29. Trovas GP, Lyritis GP, Galanos A, et al. A randomized trial of nasal spray calcitonin in men with idiopathic osteoporosis: effects on bone mineral density and bone markers. *J Bone Miner Res* 2002;17:521–7.

30. Lyritis GP, Paspati I, Karachalios T, et al. Pain relief from nasal salmon calcitonin in osteoporotic vertebral crush fractures. A double blind, placebo-controlled clinical study. *Acta Orthop Scand* 1997;275(Suppl):112–14.

31. Hamdy RC, Moore SW, Whalen KE, et al. Nandrolone decanoate for men with osteoporosis. *Am J Ther* 1998;5:89–95.

32. Behre HM, von Eckardstein S, Kliesch S, et al. Long-term substitution therapy of hypogonadal men with trans-scrotal testosterone over 7–10 years. *Clin Endocrinol* 1999;50:629–35.

33. Anderson FH, Francis RM, Peaston RT, et al. Androgen supplementation in eugonadal men with osteoporosis – effects of six months' treatment on markers of bone formation and resorption. *J Bone Miner Res* 1997;12:472–8.

34. Reid IR, Wattie DJ, Evans MC, et al. Testosterone therapy in glucocorticoid-treated men. *Arch Intern Med* 1996;156:1173–7.

35. Neer RM, Arnaud CD, Zanchetta JR, et al. Effect of parathyroid hormone (1-34) on fractures and bone mineral density in postmenopausal women with osteoporosis. *N Engl J Med* 2001;344:1434–41.

36. Kurland ES, Cosman F, McMahon DJ, et al. Parathyroid hormone as a therapy for idiopathic osteoporosis in men: effects on bone mineral density and bone markers. *J Clin Endocrinol Metab* 2000;85:3069–76.

37. Orwoll ES, Scheele WH, Paul S, et al. The effect of teriparatide [human parathyroid hormone (1-34)] therapy on bone density in men with osteoporosis. *J Bone Miner Res* 2003;18:9–17.

38. Orwoll ES, Oviatt SK, McClung MR, et al. The rate of bone mineral loss in normal men and the effects of calcium and cholecalciferol supplementation. *Ann Intern Med* 1990;112:29–34.

39. Dawson-Hughes B, Harris SS, Krall EA, et al. Effect of calcium and vitamin D supplementation on bone density in men and women 65 years of age and older. *N Engl J Med* 1997;337:670–6.

40. Trivedi DP, Doll R, Khaw KT. Effect of four monthly oral vitamin D3 (cholecalciferol) supplementation on fractures and mortality in men and women living in the community: randomised double blind controlled trial. *BMJ* 2003;326:469.

41. Ebeling PR, Wark JD, Yeung S, et al. Effects of calcitriol or calcium on bone mineral density, bone turnover and fractures in men with primary osteoporosis: a two year randomised, double blind, double placebo study. *J Clin Endocrinol Metab* 2001;86:4098–103.

42. Ringe JD, Dorst A, Kipshoven C, et al. Avoidance of vertebral fractures in men with idiopathic osteoporosis by a three year therapy with calcium and low-dose intermittent monofluorophosphate. *Osteoporos Int* 1998;8:47–52.

43. National Osteoporosis Society. Fundamentals of bone densitometry – report of a working party. Bath: National Osteoporosis Society, 1998.

44. Cummings SR, Palermo L, Browner W, et al. Monitoring osteoporosis therapy with bone densitometry: misleading changes and regression to the mean. Fracture Intervention Trial Research Group. *JAMA* 2000;283:1318–21.

45. Eastell R, Bainbridge PR. Bone turnover markers for monitoring antiresorptive therapy. *Osteoporos Rev* 2001;9:1–5.

9

Corticosteroid-induced Osteoporosis

Jackie Clowes and Richard Eastell

Introduction

Harvey Cushing first described the effect of excess corticosteroids in 1932, when he described the characteristic fracture pattern involving the pelvis, vertebrae, and ribs due to endogenous hypercortisolism. Corticosteroids remain a key component in the management of many inflammatory disorders; however, the adverse consequences, especially on bone, can be devastating. The incidence of corticosteroid-induced osteoporosis (CIO) may be as high as 50% after 6 months' treatment with steroids, and results in a 30–400% increase in the incidence of low-trauma fractures. In addition, the increase in fracture risk occurs early after the onset of therapy. Despite the availability of effective therapies, the prevalence of concomitant prescriptions of bone-active drugs for the prevention and treatment of CIO in the UK remains low.

There are many unanswered questions relating to the pathogenesis and clinical management of CIO. These include identification of the optimum bone mineral density (BMD) threshold at which to intervene with bone-active drugs, and the dose or duration of exposure to steroid therapy that warrants intervention. In addition, although many bone-active drugs prevent bone loss due to corticosteroids, data demonstrating fracture prevention are limited. The key points in CIO are summarized in **Table 9.1**. This chapter includes the National Osteoporosis Society and Royal College of Physicians guidelines [1].

Pathogenesis of corticosteroid-induced osteoporosis

Cellular effects

Corticosteroids have consistently been shown to decrease bone formation. Histomorphometry studies generally identify a reduction in bone formation, with evidence of a decrease in osteoid thickness, reduced mineral apposition rate, reduced rate of bone mineralization, and decreased osteoblast activity. The effect on bone resorption is more variable and

1% of the adult population in the UK use oral corticosteroids
After 6 months' treatment with corticosteroids, 50% of subjects may have CIO
Bone loss is early (up to 30% in 6 months) and is greatest at trabecular sites (pelvis, vertebrae, and ribs)
The rate of bone loss with long-term corticosteroid use is 2–3 times greater than that observed in age-related or postmenopausal subjects
Loss of bone density is strongly correlated with cumulative corticosteroid dose
There is a 30–400% increase in the incidence of low-trauma fractures, which is only partially reversed on stopping corticosteroid therapy
Fracture risk is correlated with cumulative and daily corticosteroid dose
A 1 standard deviation decrease in BMD results in a greater increase in fracture risk compared with an equivalent change in BMD in postmenopausal women
Fractures occur at a higher threshold in CIO compared with postmenopausal osteoporosis
Current treatment guidelines for the prevention and treatment of CIO recommend the use of a T-score cut-off of –1.5 standard deviations for BMD measurements
Treatment for CIO is cost-effective

Table 9.1 Key points in corticosteroid-induced osteoporosis (CIO). BMD: bone mineral density.

controversial. Corticosteroids can result in changes in bone strength through both trabecular thinning and, possibly, loss of trabecular connectivity, although the latter may be dose dependent [2].

The effects on bone formation appear to involve a combination of [3,4]:

- alterations in osteoblast cell differentiation
- inhibition of osteoblast matrix synthesis
- increase in osteoblast apoptosis
- modulation of gene expression

The effects of corticosteroids on osteoclasts are inconsistent, but they appear to increase osteoclast formation from bone marrow precursors and increase osteoclast apoptosis [4]. The combination of inhibition of osteoblastogenesis and increased apoptosis of osteoblasts and osteoclasts is important in CIO [5].

Different corticosteroid preparations may operate via different cellular mechanisms. The relative therapeutic advantage of the different genomic versus nongenomic potencies of corticosteroids and the impact on bone metabolism require further evaluation [6]. An enzyme, 11β-hydroxysteroid dehydrogenase type 1 (11β-HSD1), in human osteoblasts converts inactive cortisone (or prednisone) to active cortisol (or prednisolone) and may regulate glucocorticoid action [7].

Sex hormones and calcium homeostasis

Other factors that may contribute to the pathogenesis of CIO include a vitamin D-independent reduction in calcium absorption from the gastrointestinal tract, and an increase in renal calcium excretion. There is little evidence for a role of altered vitamin D metabolism, since prospective studies have failed to demonstrate any change in 25-hydroxyvitamin D_3 (25[OH]D_3) or vitamin D-binding protein [3,8]. In addition, levels of parathyroid hormone (PTH) are not consistently elevated, although corticosteroids may result in an altered renal and osteoblast sensitivity to PTH. Corticosteroids result in an acute and chronic reduction of testosterone in men; in women, high-dose steroids result in oligomenorrhea [8]. Corticosteroids mediate the effect on the reproductive hormones via an indirect effect on gonadotropins, growth hormone, and insulin-like growth factor-binding proteins, and a direct effect on the adrenal glands and gonads.

Epidemiology

The use of exogenous corticosteroids accounts for approximately 25% of osteoporosis cases and results in a significant increase in fracture risk, especially vertebral fractures in men [9]. One recent retrospective study in the UK suggests that 0.9% of the general practice population is currently using >2.5 mg/day oral corticosteroids. This extrapolates in the UK to 350,000 patients at risk of CIO; however, a concomitant prescription of a bone-active drug only occurred in approximately 5% of this population [10]. Furthermore, the use of corticosteroids was highest in the 70–79 years age group and these patients were also more likely to be prescribed a higher dose (>7.5 mg/day) for longer periods of time (>2 years) [10]. This population is especially at risk of fractures pertaining to age-related and/or postmenopausal osteoporosis, and should be regarded as an especially vulnerable group.

Effect on bone mineral density

Corticosteroid therapy results in a rapid loss in BMD; the rate of loss is greatest in the first year of therapy and may be as high as 30% in the first 6 months [8]. The accelerated rates of bone loss continue at 2–3 times higher than age-related or postmenopausal rates of bone loss, even in chronic corticosteroid therapy [11,12]. The bone loss is greatest at trabecular sites and results in fractures involving the pelvis, vertebrae, and ribs, which are characteristic of endogenous hypercortisolism or Cushing's syndrome [13]. Some studies have attempted to examine the relative contribution of the underlying disease and corticosteroids to bone loss; however, since treatment is usually prescribed to those with more severe active disease, there is always a confounding effect on bone loss.

There is some evidence that the effect on BMD is reversed on cessation of corticosteroid therapy, at least in part [14]. This is supported by the observation that patients cured of Cushing's syndrome have a normal age-matched BMD. A meta-analysis suggests that there is a strong correlation between cumulative corticosteroid dose and loss of BMD [15]. In this study, the effects of corticosteroids were not influenced by patient age or sex, although several smaller studies have reported conflicting results [15]. There does appear to be an individual heterogeneity in the response to corticosteroids, although the factors that influence the response remain unclear.

Effect on fracture risk

The use of exogenous corticosteroids results in a significant increase in fracture risk, especially vertebral fractures in men [9]. One prospective study demonstrated that oral steroids increased the relative risk of hip fracture by 80%, and by 110% after adjusting for age, rheumatoid arthritis, weight change, and femoral neck BMD [16]. Previous steroid use in men increased the risk of multiple vertebral deformities by 130% after adjusting for age [17]. Other case-control studies have suggested that the risk of hip, humeral, and distal forearm fractures is doubled in rheumatoid arthritis [18,19]. However, in a large retrospective cohort study there did not appear to be an effect of age, sex, or underlying disease on fracture [20].

A recent retrospective cohort study using the UK's General Practitioner Research Database (GPRD) demonstrated a strong correlation between daily oral corticosteroid dose and fracture risk [20]. There was also a weaker correlation between cumulative corticosteroid dose and the risk of fracture. The rate of clinical vertebral fractures increased by 55% for a prednisolone dose of <2.5 mg/day, but increased by 400% at a prednisolone dose of >7.5 mg/day. Hip, forearm, and nonvertebral fractures also displayed a dose-dependent increase in fracture risk with prednisolone doses >2.5 mg/day [20].

The incidence of nonvertebral fractures stratified by daily corticosteroid dose, age, and gender is shown in **Figure 9.1**. In a large meta-analysis, there was no statistically significant correlation with either daily or cumulative dose of corticosteroids and fracture [15]. The difference in the GPRD and meta-analysis results may arise, in part, because the GPRD study involved retrospective data from patients who were mainly using intermittent corticosteroids, whereas the meta-analysis data involved patients using continuous corticosteroids. A more recent, population-based study demonstrated an association between cumulative dose and fracture [21].

There is a rapid increase in fracture risk in the first 12 months after starting corticosteroids – an effect that is particularly marked for vertebral fractures [15]. The GPRD study also demonstrated the first evidence of a rapid decline in fracture incidence on cessation of oral corticosteroid use, especially with vertebral fractures (**Figure 9.2**). The relative fracture rate reduced from a 55% excess risk to a 25% excess risk by 12 months, although a 20% excess risk remained for at least 48 months after cessation of corticosteroid therapy (**Figure 9.3**) [20].

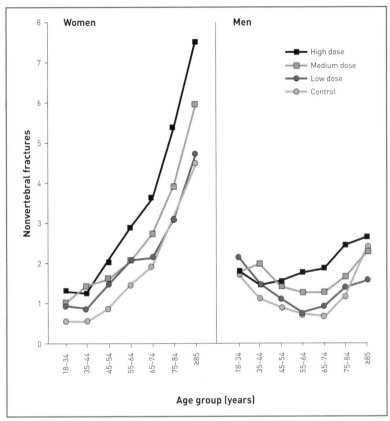

Figure 9.1 The incidence of nonvertebral fractures stratified by corticosteroid dose, age, and gender in a retrospective case-controlled study of 244,235 oral corticosteroid users. The three categories of oral corticosteroid used were low (<2.5 mg/day), medium (2.5–7.5 mg/day), and high (>7.5 mg/day) dose. Reproduced from *J Bone Miner Res* 2000;15:993–1000 with permission of the American Society for Bone and Mineral Research [20].

Effect on bone turnover markers

Osteoblastic activity may be monitored noninvasively by measuring enzymes or matrix proteins released during bone formation. In both acute and chronic use of corticosteroids, there is a dose-dependent decrease in osteocalcin, which is rapid and reversible [22,23]. The osteocalcin gene has multiple binding sites for the corticosteroid receptor, which negatively regulates the genes and provides a molecular basis for the observed effects of corticosteroids [24]. Osteocalcin appears to be especially sensitive to the systemic effects of oral, inhaled, and intra-articular corticosteroids [22,25–27]. The effect of corticosteroids on other bone formation markers suggests a suppression in measurements assessed using

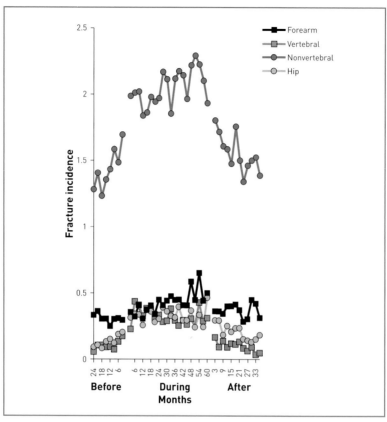

Figure 9.2 The incidence of forearm, vertebral, nonvertebral, and hip fracture before, during, and after oral corticosteroid treatment in a retrospective case-controlled study of 244,235 subjects. Reproduced from *J Bone Miner Res* 2000;15:993–1000 with permission of the American Society for Bone and Mineral Research [20].

total alkaline phosphatase (AP), procollagen type I carboxy-propeptide, and, probably, bone-specific AP [25–31]. The conversion of inactive cortisone (or prednisone) to active cortisol (or prednisolone) is regulated by the enzyme 11βHSD1 in human osteoblasts. The activity of the enzyme correlates with bone formation markers and may explain, at least in part, individual patient susceptibility to CIO [7].

Osteoclastic activity can be monitored noninvasively by measuring enzymes or matrix degradation products released during bone resorption. No consistent increases or decreases have been found in specific resorption markers in response to corticosteroids [25–31].

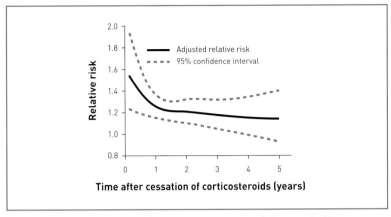

Figure 9.3 The adjusted relative risk (and 95% confidence interval) of nonvertebral fracture after discontinuation of oral corticosteroid treatment in a retrospective case-controlled study of 244,235 subjects. Reproduced from *J Bone Miner Res* 2000;15:993–1000 with permission of the American Society for Bone and Mineral Research [20].

Who should be evaluated and treated?

The clinical evaluation of CIO in individual patients involves confirmation of the diagnosis using BMD, modification of diagnostic thresholds by clinical risk factors for individual patients, investigation of underlying causes of osteoporosis, and the evaluation of problems relating to patients' activities of daily living. Guidelines on the evaluation of patients using, or expected to use, corticosteroids for >3 months are summarized in **Figure 9.4**.

Route, duration, and dose of corticosteroid therapy

The dose dependence of prednisolone-induced fractures and the increased risk of vertebral fractures, even for doses <2.5 mg/day, suggest that there is no 'safe dose' of oral corticosteroids [20]. The identification of a 'safe dose' for inhaled and nasal corticosteroids is even more difficult to evaluate [32,33].

It is generally accepted that doses >800 μg/day of beclomethasone dipropionate (BDP) or its equivalent will result in changes in BMD and adrenal suppression in adults [32]. A retrospective, population-based study found that the fracture risks in subjects using either inhaled corticosteroids or bronchodilator drugs were equivalent, although there was a small increase compared with controls [34]. This suggests that the increased fracture risk observed relates to the underlying respiratory disease, rather than the use of inhaled corticosteroids. The increase in the relative rate of fracture observed was small for nonvertebral (15%), forearm (13%), hip (22%), and vertebral (51%) fractures [34]. A small dose–response effect was observed for nonvertebral fractures, with a rate of 11% (<300 μg/day of BDP) rising to a maximum fracture rate of 28% (>700 μg/day

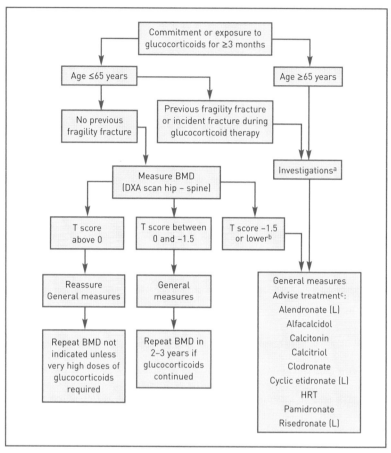

Figure 9.4 Management of corticosteroid-induced osteoporosis in men and women [1].
A fragility fracture is defined as a fracture occurring with minimum trauma after the age
of 40 years, and includes forearm, spine, hip, ribs, and pelvis.
aInvestigations in patients with previous fragility fractures (see **Table 9.2**).
bConsider treatment depending on age and fracture probability.
cTreatments listed in alphabetic order.
Vitamin D and calcium are generally regarded as adjuncts to treatment. Hormone replacement
therapy (HRT) comprises estrogen in postmenopausal women and testosterone in men.
(L) indicates that the drug is licensed for corticosteroid-induced osteoporosis.
BMD: bone mineral density; DXA: dual-energy X-ray absorptiometry.

of BDP). A statistically significant increase in hip (77%) and vertebral (150%)
fractures was only observed at BDP doses >700 µg/day [34].

Certain inhaled and oral corticosteroids, eg, budesonide and deflazacort,
have been reported as bone sparing. However, uncertainty about the relative

anti-inflammatory potency of different preparations and the small sample sizes used in the majority of comparative studies mean that it is not possible to make specific recommendations on the relative benefits of different corticosteroids.

The duration of corticosteroid use by patients varies depending on the disease process, severity, and natural history. A retrospective, population-based study found that 19% of patients with musculoskeletal disease continued treatment for >2 years compared with 6% of patients with respiratory disease [10]. It is important to emphasize that cessation of corticosteroid therapy results in a rapid reversal of nonvertebral fracture risk by 12 months, although the reduction in the excess risk of fracture is only partially reversed on stopping treatment [20]. A similar partial reversal of excess risk was seen with inhaled corticosteroids [34]. It is therefore important that clinicians evaluate patients' fracture risk early and consider the need for corticosteroid treatment for more than a few months.

Evaluation of clinical risk factors

Prospective studies of hip fractures in postmenopausal women have identified independent risk factors including age, sex, Caucasian race, a history of prevalent fracture, recurrent falls, family history of fracture, and health status. These risk factors have never been evaluated in relation to fracture risk in CIO, although it is sensible to consider them when assessing an individual's fracture risk. Models need to be developed to assess the absolute risk of fracture based on combinations of readily ascertainable risk factors and BMD in CIO.

Separating the contribution of the drug therapy from the disease process as a confounding factor remains very difficult. The clinical conditions that most frequently require treatment with corticosteroid therapy may themselves have a direct effect on bone density and fracture risk [10]. The most frequent indications for oral corticosteroid use are respiratory (40%), skin (6%), musculoskeletal (6%), neurologic (3%), and gastrointestinal (3%) disorders. One important cause of fractures is solid organ transplantation, with an estimated increased relative risk of 5- to 34-fold, depending on patient gender and the type of transplantation. In a case-control study, chronic respiratory disease in women was associated with a 3-fold increase in severe vertebral deformities; this remained significant, despite correcting for corticosteroid use. However, in a large retrospective cohort study, there did not appear to be an effect of age, gender, or underlying disease on fracture risk [20].

Diagnostic threshold for bone mineral density

It has been suggested that patients with CIO develop fractures at a higher threshold of BMD than age-related or postmenopausal osteoporosis [35], although a more recent study did not confirm this [36]. It is important to note that, in the former study, patients using corticosteroids were more likely to have multiple fractures, despite an equivalent T-score at the lumbar spine, which might suggest that there is reduced bone quality in CIO [36]. In addition, it is generally accepted that a 1 standard deviation (SD) decrease in BMD results in

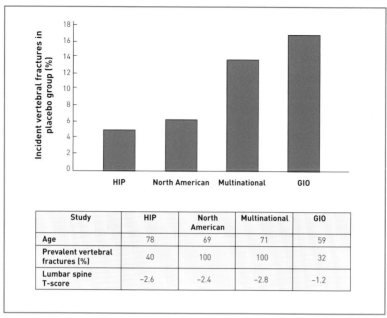

Figure 9.5 The percentage of incident vertebral fractures (graph), and age, prevalent fractures, and T-scores (table) for three randomized controlled trials in postmenopausal osteoporosis versus corticosteroid-induced osteoporosis, demonstrating a difference in 'fracture threshold'. GIO: glucocorticoid-induced osteoporosis; HIP: Hip Intervention Program. Adapted from [39–42].

a doubling of fracture risk in postmenopausal women [37]. However, in postmenopausal women using corticosteroids for rheumatoid arthritis, there was a 6-fold increased risk of vertebral fractures, with a decrease in BMD of <1 SD at the lumbar spine [38].

A strong case for a different 'fracture threshold' in CIO compared with postmenopausal osteoporosis can be made by reviewing the vertebral fracture rate in the placebo group of several randomized controlled trials (RCTs) [39–42]. The data demonstrate a higher lumbar spine T-score of –1.2 in the CIO study compared with –2.4 to –2.8 in the postmenopausal osteoporosis (Hip Intervention Program, North American, and multinational vertebral) studies (**Figure 9.5**) [39–42].

Despite the higher lumbar spine T-score, there was a dramatically higher percentage (16%) of incident vertebral fractures in the placebo arm of the CIO study compared with the postmenopausal osteoporosis studies (5–13%). These differences occurred despite the greater average age and higher prevalent vertebral fracture rate in the postmenopausal osteoporosis studies.

In patients with previous fragility fractures:

- Full blood count and erythrocyte sedimentation rate
- Bone and liver function tests (calcium, phosphate, alkaline phosphatase, albumin, alanine transferase, γ-glutamyl transferase)
- Serum creatinine
- Serum thyroid-stimulating hormone

If indicated:

- Lateral thoracic and lumbar spine X-rays
- Serum paraproteins and urine Bence–Jones protein
- Isotope bone scan
- Serum follicle-stimulating hormone if hormone status unclear (women)
- Serum testosterone, luteinizing hormone, and sex hormone-binding globulin (men)
- Serum parathyroid hormone and 25-hydroxyvitamin D
- BMD if monitoring required

Table 9.2 Investigations in patients with previous fragility fractures [1]. BMD: bone mineral density.

These factors represent independent risk factors for incident fractures and would therefore be expected to increase the incident fracture rate in the postmenopausal osteoporosis studies.

A UK consensus group recommended the use of a T-score cut-off of −1.5 SD for central densitometry measurements in assessing subjects for the prevention and treatment of CIO compared with a T-score cut-off of −1.0 SD from the American College of Rheumatology [1,43]. However, the appropriate BMD threshold for intervention and the relative risk of fracture for every 1 SD decrease in BMD in patients using corticosteroids still require further evaluation. The absence of high-quality evidence of the BMD threshold appropriate to initiate treatment in CIO is reflected in the wide diversity of intervention thresholds used by rheumatologists in clinical practice [44].

In addition, diagnostic thresholds in CIO have not been determined for peripheral densitometry using either dual-energy X-ray absorptiometry or quantitative ultrasound. Therefore, these technologies should currently be used with caution when assessing fracture risk. A cost-effectiveness analysis in female patients starting corticosteroid therapy for rheumatoid arthritis suggests a cost of $76,100 per quality of adjusted life years using a T-score of less than −2.5 SD [45]. However, this analysis severely underestimated the fracture rates in CIO, and a reanalysis using more robust fracture data would be valuable [20].

Laboratory evaluation

The utility of testing for secondary causes of osteoporosis in CIO has not been studied in men or women. Therefore, recommendations on which groups of patients to evaluate and the appropriate investigations to perform are based on clinical experience. The most likely etiologic factor is the use of corticosteroids. However, patients presenting with unusual clinical features and all patients with a low-trauma vertebral fracture probably warrant laboratory evaluation for secondary causes of osteoporosis (**Table 9.2**).

A general evaluation should include measurement of calcium, phosphate, renal and liver function, AP, full blood count, erythrocyte sedimentation rate, thyroid-stimulating hormone (hyperthyroidism), PTH (primary and secondary hyperparathyroidism), serum and urine immunoelectrophoresis (myeloma), and testosterone, sex hormone-binding globulin, and follicle-stimulating hormone in all men (hypogonadism). Other investigations to consider include lateral thoracic and lumbar X-rays and an isotope bone scan.

Drug therapy in children, premenopausal women, and men

The majority of data on the effect of corticosteroids on bone loss or fracture risk are derived from studies of postmenopausal women. It is important to remember in premenopausal women (and children) that the absolute fracture risk is low. The current National Osteoporosis Society and Royal College of Physicians guidelines suggest that prophylaxis against bone loss should be restricted to those with very low BMD with or without the presence of fragility fractures or other strong risk factors [1]. It is important to consider the use of bisphosphonates in premenopausal women with great caution, as they cross the placenta and teratogenic effects have been observed in animal studies [1].

Small studies in men have demonstrated the prevention of corticosteroid-induced bone loss. However, except in elderly men, the fracture risk is low. In children, the majority of data are derived from the use of pamidronate in osteogenesis imperfecta.

What are the treatment options?

The majority of studies on the effects of drug treatment in patients using corticosteroids have examined bone loss as the primary endpoint, with the effect on vertebral or nonvertebral fractures as a secondary endpoint or as part of safety monitoring (**Table 9.3**).

Lifestyle modification and falls assessment

Recommendations on lifestyle modification, falls assessment, and falls prevention are largely based on observational studies and RCTs in postmenopausal women, and have not been evaluated in CIO. It is, however, reasonable to assume a similar impact when assessing fracture risk and prevention of CIO. Interestingly, a meta-regression analysis of drug treatment for CIO suggested that vitamin D

Therapeutic intervention	Outcome measure			
	Spine BMD	Hip BMD	Vertebral fractures	Nonvertebral fractures
Calcium, vitamin D, and vitamin D metabolites				
Calcium	nd	nd	–	–
Calcium + vitamin D	A[b]	A[b]	–	–
Calcitriol	A[b]	A[b]	–	nd
Alfacalcidol	A	A[b]	–	nd
Bisphosphonates				
Alendronate	A	A	A[a]	A[a]
Clodronate	A	A	–	–
Etidronate	A	A	A[a]	A[a]
Pamidronate	A	A	–	–
Risedronate	A	A	A[a]	A[a]
Sex hormones				
HRT or Tibolone	A	A	–	–
Raloxifene	–	–	–	–
Testosterone (men)	A	–	–	–
Others				
PTH	A	A	–	–
Calcitonin	A[b]	A[b]	nd	nd
Fluoride	A	nd	–	–

Table 9.3 Recommendations and evidence for treatment in corticosteroid-induced osteoporosis. Grading of recommendations and evidence levels: Grade A: meta-analysis of randomized controlled trials or at least one adequately powered randomized controlled trial; Grade B: at least one well-designed, controlled study without randomization, comparative study, or case-controlled study; Grade C: expert opinion.
[a]Not a primary endpoint.
[b]Data inconsistent.
BMD: bone mineral density; HRT: hormone replacement therapy; nd: no effect detected; not adequately assessed or no data; PTH: parathyroid hormone. Adapted from [1,7].

enhanced the effectiveness of bisphosphonates on bone density measurements [46]. In all patients using corticosteroids, it is important to optimize calcium and vitamin D intake and consider lifestyle modifications, eg, maintaining exercise levels (**Table 9.4**).

Calcium, vitamin D, and vitamin D metabolites
A meta-analysis compared RCTs involving 274 subjects randomized to either vitamin D (cholecalciferol) or dihydroxyvitamin D (calcitriol) with calcium

General measures
Reduce dose of corticosteroids when possible
Consider corticosteroid-sparing therapy, eg, azathioprine, if appropriate
Consider alternative route of glucocorticoid administration
Lifestyle measures
Recommend good nutrition, especially with adequate calcium and vitamin D
Recommend regular weight-bearing exercise
Maintain body weight
Avoid tobacco use and alcohol abuse
Assess falls risk and give appropriate advice

Table 9.4 General and lifestyle measures in the management of corticosteroid-induced osteoporosis [1].

versus calcium alone or placebo. This identified a statistically significant weighted mean difference (WMD) for vitamin or dihydroxyvitamin D with calcium of 2.6 (95% confidence interval [CI] 0.7–4.5) at the lumbar spine and 2.5 (95% CI 0.6–4.4) at the radius, but not at the femoral neck (0.4 [95% CI −1.1–1.8) [47]. It is important to note that a WMD identifies the difference between treatment and control and does not necessarily reflect an absolute gain in BMD. The incidence of nontraumatic fractures was not significant, with a summary odds ratio of 0.6 (95% CI 0.1– 2.4) [47]. More recent studies have provided similar results [48–50].

Bisphosphonates

A substantial body of evidence has demonstrated the efficacy of bisphosphonates in the prevention and treatment of bone loss and in fracture prevention [1,41,46,51–59]. For example, risedronate has been shown to reduce vertebral fractures by 70% at 1 year compared with placebo in men and women treated with corticosteroids [41,60]. In addition, vitamin D may enhance the effectiveness of bisphosphonate therapy [46].

Sex steroid hormones

The role of hormone replacement therapy (HRT) in the prevention or treatment of CIO or fractures is based on a limited number of studies. In studies of patients using corticosteroids for the treatment of either asthma or rheumatoid arthritis, there was a significant increase in BMD at the lumbar spine in patients using HRT compared with no treatment or calcium alone [61,62]. Tibolone has recently been shown to prevent bone loss in subjects using corticosteroids for rheumatoid arthritis [63]. Testosterone in men has been shown to prevent bone loss at the lumbar spine in CIO [64].

Parathyroid hormone

One study examined the effect of 12 months' treatment with PTH in postmenopausal women already using HRT and corticosteroids. There was an 11% increase in lumbar spine BMD with PTH compared with HRT alone. No difference was observed at either the hip or forearm. During the subsequent 12 months without PTH, the treatment benefit was maintained at the lumbar spine, and the hip BMD was significantly increased compared with those receiving HRT alone [65].

Calcitonin

A meta-analysis of RCTs involving 441 subjects randomized to either calcitonin or placebo has been published [67]. This identified a statistically significant WMD of 3.2 (95% CI 0.3–6.1) at the lumbar spine by 12 months, which was no longer significant by 24 months (4.5 [95% CI –0.6–9.5]) for the active treatment group. The results were not significant at the radius or femoral neck at 12 or 24 months [66]. The relative risk of vertebral fractures was reduced to 0.71 (95% CI 0.26–1.89) and nonvertebral fractures to 0.52 (95% CI 0.14–1.96), but neither reached statistical significance [66].

Conclusion

The increase in fracture risk with corticosteroids occurs early after the onset of therapy, and there appears to be no 'safe' treatment dose. In addition, there is only a partial reversal of bone loss and fracture risk on cessation of therapy. It is therefore important that clinicians evaluate patients' fracture risk early and consider the need for the prevention and treatment of bone loss and fractures in all patients using corticosteroids for more than a few months.

References

1. Compston JE, Barlow D, Brown P, et al. *Glucocorticoid-induced Osteoporosis; Guidelines for Prevention and Treatment*. London: Royal College of Physicians, 2002:1–57.

2. Dalle Carbonare L, Arlot ME, Chavassieux PM, et al. Comparison of trabecular bone microarchitecture and remodeling in glucocorticoid-induced and postmenopausal osteoporosis. *J Bone Miner Res* 2001;16:97–103.

3. Manolagas SC, Weinstein RS. New developments in the pathogenesis and treatment of steroid-induced osteoporosis. *J Bone Miner Res* 1999;14:1061–6.

4. Bland R. Steroid hormone receptor expression and action in bone. *Clin Sci (Lond)* 2000;98:217–40.

5. Weinstein RS, Jilka RL, Parfitt AM, et al. Inhibition of osteoblastogenesis and promotion of apoptosis of osteoblasts and osteocytes by glucocorticoids. Potential mechanisms of their deleterious effects on bone. *J Clin Invest* 1998;102:274–82.

6. Lipworth BJ. Therapeutic implications of non-genomic glucocorticoid activity. *Lancet* 2000;356:87–9.

7. Cooper MS, Blumsohn A, Goddard PE, et al. 11beta-hydroxysteroid dehydrogenase type 1 activity predicts the effects of glucocorticoids on bone. *J Clin Endocrinol Metab* 2003;88:3874–7.

8. Reid IR. Glucocorticoid-induced osteoporosis. *Baillieres Best Pract Res Clin Endocrinol Metab* 2000;14:279–98.

9. Eastell R, Reid DM, Compston J, et al. A UK Consensus Group on management of glucocorticoid-induced osteoporosis: an update. *J Intern Med* 1998;244:271–92.

10. van Staa TP, Leufkens HG, Abenhaim L, et al. Use of oral corticosteroids in the United Kingdom. *QJM* 2000;93:105–11.

11. Gennari C, Pollavini G, Nami R, et al. Influence of intravenous beta-adrenergic blockade with or without partial agonist activity upon plasma cyclic AMP and catecholamines in healthy subjects. *Eur J Clin Pharmacol* 1984;26:695–8.

12. Saito JK, Davis JW, Wasnich RD, et al. Users of low-dose glucocorticoids have increased bone loss rates: a longitudinal study. *Calcif Tissue Int* 1995;57:115–19.

13. Freehill AK, Lenke LG. Severe kyphosis secondary to glucocorticoid-induced osteoporosis in a young adult with Cushing's disease. A case report and literature review. *Spine* 1999;24:189–93.

14. Laan RF, van Riel PL, van de Putte LB, et al. Low-dose prednisone induces rapid reversible axial bone loss in patients with rheumatoid arthritis. A randomized, controlled study. *Ann Intern Med* 1993;119:963–8.

15. van Staa TP, Leufkens HG, Cooper C. The epidemiology of corticosteroid-induced osteoporosis: a meta-analysis. *Osteoporos Int* 2002;13:777–87.

16. Baltzan MA, Suissa S, Bauer DC, et al. Hip fractures attributable to corticosteroid use. Study of Osteoporotic Fractures Group. *Lancet* 1999;353:1327.

17. Ismail AA, O'Neill TW, Cooper C, et al. Risk factors for vertebral deformities in men: relationship to number of vertebral deformities. European Vertebral Osteoporosis Study Group. *J Bone Miner Res* 2000;15:278–83.

18. Hooyman JR, Melton LJ III, Nelson AM, et al. Fractures after rheumatoid arthritis. A population-based study. *Arthritis Rheum* 1984;27:1353–61.

19. Cooper C, Coupland C, Mitchell M. Rheumatoid arthritis, corticosteroid therapy and hip fracture. *Ann Rheum Dis* 1995;54:49–52.

20. van Staa TP, Leufkens HG, Abenhaim L, et al. Use of oral corticosteroids and risk of fractures. *J Bone Miner Res* 2000;15:993–1000.

21. Walsh LJ, Lewis SA, Wong CA, et al. The impact of oral corticosteroid use on bone mineral density and vertebral fracture. *Am J Respir Crit Care Med* 2002;166:691–5.

22. Cosman F, Nieves J, Herbert J, et al. High-dose glucocorticoids in multiple sclerosis patients exert direct effects on the kidney and skeleton. *J Bone Miner Res* 1994;9:1097–105.

23. Godschalk MF, Downs RW. Effect of short-term glucocorticoids on serum osteocalcin in healthy young men. *J Bone Miner Res* 1988;3:113–15.

24. Morrison NA, Shine J, Fragonas JC, et al. 1,25-dihydroxyvitamin D-responsive element and glucocorticoid repression in the osteocalcin gene. *Science* 1989;246:1158–61.

25. Prummel MF, Wiersinga WM, Lips P, et al. The course of biochemical parameters of bone turnover during treatment with corticosteroids. *J Clin Endocrinol Metab* 1991;72:382–6.

26. Lems WF, Gerrits MI, Jacobs JW, et al. Changes in (markers of) bone metabolism during high dose corticosteroid pulse treatment in patients with rheumatoid arthritis. *Ann Rheum Dis* 1996;55:288–93.

27. Lane SJ, Vaja S, Swaminathan R, et al. Effects of prednisolone on bone turnover in patients with corticosteroid resistant asthma. *Clin Exp Allergy* 1996;26:1197–201.

28. Morrison D, Ali NJ, Routledge PA, et al. Bone turnover during short course prednisolone treatment in patients with chronic obstructive airways disease. *Thorax* 1992;47:418–20.

29. Wolthers OD. Methodological aspects of short-term knemometry in the assessment of exogenous glucocorticosteroid-induced growth suppression in children. *Ann Hum Biol* 1997;24:539–46.

30. Gonnelli S, Rottoli P, Cepollaro C, et al. Prevention of corticosteroid-induced osteoporosis with alendronate in sarcoid patients. *Calcif Tissue Int* 1997;61:382–5.

31. Pearce G, Tabensky DA, Delmas PD, et al. Corticosteroid-induced bone loss in men. *J Clin Endocrinol Metab* 1998;83:801–6.

32. Cave A, Arlett P, Lee E. Inhaled and nasal corticosteroids: factors affecting the risks of systemic adverse effects. *Pharmacol Ther* 1999;83:153–79.

33. Wong CA, Walsh LJ, Smith CJ, et al. Inhaled corticosteroid use and bone-mineral density in patients with asthma. *Lancet* 2000;355:1399–403.

34. van Staa TP, Leufkens HG, Cooper C. Use of inhaled corticosteroids and risk of fractures. *J Bone Miner Res* 2001;16:581–8.

35. Luengo M, Picado C, del Rio L, et al. Vertebral fractures in steroid dependent asthma and involutional osteoporosis: a comparative study. *Thorax* 1991;46:803–6.

36. Selby PL, Halsey JP, Adams KR, et al. Corticosteroids do not alter the threshold for vertebral fracture. *J Bone Miner Res* 2000;15:952–6.

37. Marshall D, Johnell O, Wedel H. Meta-analysis of how well measures of bone mineral density predict occurrence of osteoporotic fractures. *BMJ* 1996;312:1254–9.

38. Peel NF, Moore DJ, Barrington NA, et al. Risk of vertebral fracture and relationship to bone mineral density in steroid treated rheumatoid arthritis. *Ann Rheum Dis* 1995;54:801–6.

39. Harris ST, Watts NB, Genant HK, et al. Effects of risedronate treatment on vertebral and nonvertebral fractures in women with postmenopausal osteoporosis: a randomized controlled trial. Vertebral Efficacy With Risedronate Therapy (VERT) Study Group. *JAMA* 1999;282:1344–52.

40. Reginster J, Minne HW, Sorensen OH, et al. Randomized trial of the effects of risedronate on vertebral fractures in women with established postmenopausal osteoporosis. Vertebral Efficacy with Risedronate Therapy (VERT) Study Group. *Osteoporos Int* 2000;11:83–91.

41. Wallach S, Cohen S, Reid DM, et al. Effects of risedronate treatment on bone density and vertebral fracture in patients on corticosteroid therapy. *Calcif Tissue Int* 2000;67:277–85.

42. McClung MR, Geusens P, Miller PD, et al. Effect of risedronate on the risk of hip fracture in elderly women. Hip Intervention Program Study Group. *N Engl J Med* 2001;344:333–40.

43. Recommendations for the prevention and treatment of glucocorticoid-induced osteoporosis. American College of Rheumatology Task Force on Osteoporosis Guidelines. *Arthritis Rheum* 1996;39:1791–801.

44. Soucy E, Bellamy N, Adachi JD, et al. A Canadian survey on the management of corticosteroid induced osteoporosis by rheumatologists. *J Rheumatol* 2000;27:1506–12.

45. Solomon DH, Kuntz KM. Should postmenopausal women with rheumatoid arthritis who are starting corticosteroid treatment be screened for osteoporosis? A cost-effectiveness analysis. *Arthritis Rheum* 2000;43:1967–75.

46. Amin S, Lavalley MP, Simms RW, et al. The comparative efficacy of drug therapies used for the management of corticosteroid-induced osteoporosis: a meta-regression. *J Bone Miner Res* 2002;17:1512–26.

47. Homik J, Suarez-Almazor ME, Shea B, et al. Calcium and vitamin D for corticosteroid-induced osteoporosis. *Cochrane Database Syst Rev* 2000;CD000952.

48. Ringe JD, Coster A, Meng T, et al. Treatment of glucocorticoid-induced osteoporosis with alfacalcidol/calcium versus vitamin D/calcium. *Calcif Tissue Int* 1999;65:337–40.

49. Reginster JY, de Froidmont C, Lecart MP, et al. Alphacalcidol in prevention of glucocorticoid-induced osteoporosis. *Calcif Tissue Int* 1999;65:328–31.

50. Lakatos P, Nagy Z, Kiss L, et al. Prevention of corticosteroid-induced osteoporosis by alfacalcidol. *Z Rheumatol* 2000;59(Suppl 1):48–52.

51. Sebaldt RJ, Ioannidis G, Adachi JD, et al. 36 month intermittent cyclical etidronate treatment in patients with established corticosteroid induced osteoporosis. *J Rheumatol* 1999;26:1545–9.

52. Jenkins EA, Walker-Bone KE, Wood A, et al. The prevention of corticosteroid-induced bone loss with intermittent cyclical etidronate. *Scand J Rheumatol* 1999;28:152–6.

53. Cortet B, Hachulla E, Barton I, et al. Evaluation of the efficacy of etidronate therapy in preventing glucocorticoid-induced bone loss in patients with inflammatory rheumatic diseases. A randomized study. *Rev Rhum Engl Ed* 1999;66:214–19.

54. Cohen S, Levy RM, Keller M, et al. Risedronate therapy prevents corticosteroid-induced bone loss: a twelve-month, multicenter, randomized, double-blind, placebo-controlled, parallel-group study. *Arthritis Rheum* 1999;42:2309–18.

55. Saag KG, Emkey R, Schnitzer TJ, et al. Alendronate for the prevention and treatment of glucocorticoid-induced osteoporosis. Glucocorticoid-Induced Osteoporosis Intervention Study Group. *N Engl J Med* 1998;339:292–9.

56. Roux C, Oriente P, Laan R, et al. Randomized trial of effect of cyclical etidronate in the prevention of corticosteroid-induced bone loss. Ciblos Study Group. *J Clin Endocrinol Metab* 1998;83:1128–33.

57. Pitt P, Li F, Todd P, et al. A double blind placebo controlled study to determine the effects of intermittent cyclical etidronate on bone mineral density in patients on long-term oral corticosteroid treatment. *Thorax* 1998;53:351–6.

58. Herrala J, Puolijoki H, Liippo K, et al. Clodronate is effective in preventing corticosteroid-induced bone loss among asthmatic patients. *Bone* 1998;22:577–82.

59. Homik J, Cranney A, Shea B, et al. Bisphosphonates for steroid induced osteoporosis. *Cochrane Database Syst Rev* 2000;CD001347.

60. Reid DM, Hughes RA, Laan RF, et al. Efficacy and safety of daily risedronate in the treatment of corticosteroid-induced osteoporosis in men and women: a randomized trial. European Corticosteroid-Induced Osteoporosis Treatment Study. *J Bone Miner Res* 2000;15:1006–13.

61. Lukert BP. Glucocorticoid-induced osteoporosis. *South Med J* 1992;85:2S48–51.

62. Hall GM, Daniels M, Doyle DV, et al. Effect of hormone replacement therapy on bone mass in rheumatoid arthritis patients treated with and without steroids. *Arthritis Rheum* 1994;37:1499–505.

63. Guglielmi G, Cammisa M, De Serio A, et al. Phalangeal US velocity discriminates between normal and vertebrally fractured subjects. *Eur Radiol* 1999;9:1632–7.

64. Reid IR, Wattie DJ, Evans MC, et al. Testosterone therapy in glucocorticoid-treated men. *Arch Intern Med* 1996;156:1173–7.

65. Lane NE, Sanchez S, Modin GW, et al. Parathyroid hormone treatment can reverse corticosteroid-induced osteoporosis. Results of a randomized controlled clinical trial. *J Clin Invest* 1998;102:1627–33.

66. Cranney A, Welch V, Adachi JD, et al. Calcitonin for the treatment and prevention of corticosteroid-induced osteoporosis. *Cochrane Database Syst Rev* 2000;CD001983.

Abbreviations

11βHSD$_1$	11β-hydroxysteroid dehydrogenase type 1
1,25(OH)$_2$D$_3$	1,25-dihydroxyvitamin D$_3$
25(OH)D$_3$	25-hydroxyvitamin D$_3$
AP	alkaline phosphatase
BDP	beclomethasone dipropionate
BFR	bone formation rate
BMC	bone mineral content
BMD	bone mineral density
BMI	body mass index
BSAP	bone-specific alkaline phosphatase
BSP	bone sialoprotein
BUA	broadband ultrasonic attenuation
Cbfa	core binding factor
CEE	conjugated equine estrogens
CI	confidence interval
CIO	corticosteroid-induced osteoporosis
CM	colorimetric method
Cr	creatinine
CT	computed tomography
CTX	C-terminal telopeptide
CV	coefficient of variation
DHT	dihydrotestosterone
DPD	deoxypyridinoline
DXA	dual-energy X-ray absorptiometry
EPIDOS	Epidemiologie de l'Osteoporose study
ER	estrogen receptor
ESR	erythrocyte sedimentation rate
EVOS	European Vertebral Osteoporosis study
FICSIT	The Frailty and Injuries: Cooperative Studies of Intervention Techniques
FSH	follicle-stimulating hormone
GGHYL	glucosyl-galactosyl-hydroxylysine
GHYL	galactosyl-hydroxylysine
GLA	γ-carboxyglutamic acid
GP	general practitioner

GPRD	General Practitioner Research Database
HAL	hip axis length
HPLC	high performance liquid chromatography
HRT	hormone replacement therapy
IA	immunoassay
ICSBM	International Committee for Standards in Bone Measurement
ICTP	carboxy-terminal telopeptide of type I collagen
IGF	insulin-like growth factor
IL	interleukin
LH	luteinizing hormone
M-CSF	macrophage colony-stimulating factor
MEDOS	Mediterranean Osteoporosis Study
MORE	Multiple Outcomes of Raloxifene Evaluation study
NaF	sodium fluoride
Na_2PO_4F	monofluorophosphate
nd	not demonstrated
Nd/Lp	node-to-loop
Nd/Nd	node-to-node
Nd/Tm	node-to-terminus
NHANES	National Health and Nutrition Examination Survey
NICE	National Institute for Clinical Excellence
NOF	National Osteoporosis Foundation
NSA	neck shaft angle
NTX	N-terminal telopeptide
OC	osteocalcin
OFELY	Os des Femmes de Lyon study
OHP	hydroxyproline
OPG	osteoprotegerin
PA	posteroanterior
PBM	peak bone mass
pDXA	peripheral dual-energy X-ray absorptiometry
PICP	C-terminal propeptide of type I procollagen
PINP	N-terminal propeptide of type I procollagen
pQCT	peripheral quantitative computed tomography
pQUS	peripheral quantitative ultrasound
PROOF	Prevent Recurrence of Osteoporotic Fractures study
PTH	parathyroid hormone
PYD	pyridinoline
QCT	quantitative computed tomography
QUALEFFO	Quality of Life Questionnaire of the European Foundation for Osteoporosis
QUS	quantitative ultrasound
RA	radiographic absorptiometry
RANK	receptor activator of nuclear factor-κB
RANKL	receptor activator of nuclear factor-κB ligand

RCP	Royal College of Physicians
RCT	randomized controlled trial
rhPTH	recombinant human parathyroid hormone
ROC	receiver operating characteristic
ROI	region of interest
RR	relative risk
SARM	selective androgen receptor modulator
sBMD	standardized bone mineral density
SD	standard deviation
SERM	selective estrogen receptor modulator
SHBG	sex hormone-binding globulin
SOC	serum osteocalcin
SOF	Study of Osteoporotic Fractures
SOS	speed of sound
SOTI	Spinal Osteoporosis Therapeutic Intervention
T_3	triiodothyronine
T_4	thyroxine
TENS	transcutaneous electrical nerve stimulation
TGF	transforming growth factor
Tm/Tm	terminus-to-terminus
TNF	tumor necrosis factor
TRAP	tartrate-resistant acid phosphatase
TROPOS	Treatment of Peripheral Osteoporosis Study
TSH	thyroxine-stimulating hormone
VOS	velocity of sound
WHI	Women's Health Initiative
WHO	World Health Organization
WMD	weighted mean difference

Index

All entries refer to osteoporosis unless otherwise stated.
Entries in **bold** refer to figures.
Entries in *italics* refer to tables or boxes.

A

B

C

D